I0470645

301 NCLEX-RN Study Tips

Easy to remember study tips for Nursing school and the NCLEX-RN exam

version 2013-1

By Jim Vickery RN

This document describes ways to study for nursing school and the NCLEX-RN exam by using easy to remember study tips. Follow the easy to remember acronyms and anecdotes for better retention of information ©

Table of Contents

Chapter 1-

Endocrine System

Signs and Symptoms of Hypoglycemia:

To remember the signs and symptoms of Hypoglycemia use the word: COOL

C- Cool clammy skin
O- Overly hungry
O- Oral mucosa will be numb
L- likely to feel faint

Jaundice

Since jaundice can be caused by cirrhosis, use the word, "CIRRHOSIS" to remember the causes of jaundice use the word:

C- Cirrhosis
I- Inadequate blood flow to liver
R- Ripe - as in a congenital disorder
R- Red blood cells that are broken down
H- Hepatitis
O- Obstruction of bile duct, as from a gallstone
S- Some types of cancer, like pancreatic cancer
I- Infection from malaria
S- Stricture of bile duct

Treatment of Pheochromocytoma

Since pheochromocytoma is caused by a tumor, use TUMOR to remember the treatments for this condition.

T- Treat with prazosin (to block alpha-adrenergic activity)
U- Use of diuretics should be avoided
M- Must control blood pressure: with beta blockers
O- Operation for removal of tumor
R- Requires follow up treatment to confirm a cure

Signs and Symptoms of Urolithiasis

Since one of the first symptoms in kidney stones is a sharp pain, use the word SHARP to remember the signs and symptoms of kidney stones.

S- Sometimes nausea and vomiting

H- Hematuria

A- Acid (uric) may be seen in urine and blood tests

R- Region of pain may move to groin

P- Pain that is SHARP and cramping

Treatment of Urolithiasis

Since one of the primary goals of treatment for Urolithiasis is the removal of stones, use the word REMOVAL to remember the treatment of Urolithiasis

R- Removal of stones by either insertion of Foley catheter if bladder is obstructed

E- Esidrix – (it lowers calcium concentration)

M- May need surgery if there is an obstructed infected portion of urinary tract

O- Occurs more in men than women (Patient Teaching)

V- Vitamin intake may increase risk (Patient Teaching)

A- Allopurinol (lowers urinary uric acid)

L- Lab studies (may be helpful in identifying risk factors for stone formation)

Acute Pancreatitis Signs and Symptoms

Acute Pancreatitis is an inflammation of the pancreas. Therefore to remember the signs and symptoms of this

condition think of the word, "INFLAMED".

    I- Increased respiratory rate
    N- Nausea and vomiting
    F- Fluid volume low
    L- Low skin turgor
    A- Absent or decreased bowel sounds
    M- Mid-epigastric pain
    E- Elevated blood pressure and heart rate
    D- Distended Abdomen

Etiology of Hepatic Failure

Since the liver is involved in Hepatic failure, to remember the causes of hepatic failure use the word, LIVER.

    L- Liver disease
    I- Ingestion of toxic substances
    V- Viral hepatitis
    E- Excessive use of acetaminophen
    R- Real high use of alcohol

Signs and Symptoms of Hepatic Failure

To remember the signs and symptoms of Hepatic Failure use the word, FAILURE.

F- Failure of the renal system
A- Asterixis (flapping of the wrists)
I- Increased heart rate
L- Labored respirations
U- unsightly jaundice
R- Respiratory rate is high
E- Ecchymosis

Treatment of Hepatic Failure

To remember the treatments of hepatic failure use the word, VITAMIN.

V- Vitamin K (as ordered)
I- Institute bleeding precautions
T- Turn every 2 hours
A- Administer potassium (as ordered)
M- Monitor for shock
I- In patients with ascites, diuretics my be needed
N- Note any dyspnea or cough which could indicate pulmonary edema

Signs and Symptoms of DKA

Diabetic Ketoacidosis is characterized by hyperglycemia, acidosis and ketones. Since of the symptoms of DKA is a fruity breath, to remember the signs and symptoms use the word, FRUITY

> F- Fruity acetone breath
> R- Respirations are deep and rapid
> U- Urine will have ketones
> I- Increase in glucose (usually greater than 300 mg/dl)
> T- Tremors may be present
> Y- Yes, there will be hypotension

Treatments of DKA

To remember the treatments of DKA, think of the word of the medication that is used to treat it, namely, INSULIN.

I- Insulin (to lower the glucose levels)
N- Nutrition
S- Small frequent meals
U- Unconscious patient will require body
   alignment to be maintained
L- Loss of potassium will require potassium
   chloride (as ordered)
I- IV infusions of insulin
N- Need to cough and deep breath the conscious
   patient to prevent pulmonary stasis

Hyperglycemia without DKA

To remember the signs and symptoms of this condition use the phrase, "NO KETOSIS" since no ketosis is involved in this situation.

N- No ketosis or acidosis
O- Older population is often affected

K- Kussmauls respirations will not occur
E- Excessive urine (polyuria)
T- Thirst will be excessive (polydipsia)
O- Orthostatic hypotension
S- Seizures may occur
I- Increased respirations
S- Signs of hemiparesis

Signs and Symptoms of Hypoglycemia

Hypoglycemia is a condition of low glucose levels that results in wet skin. Therefore, to remember the signs and symptoms of hypoglycemia think of the words, "WET SKIN".

W- Wet skin (i.e., diaphoresis)
E- Extreme hunger
T- Tachycardia

S- Skin is cool to the touch
K- Ketones in blood serum is negative
I- Inability to concentrate
N- Numbness of tongue and lips

Treatment of Hypoglycemia

To remember the treatment of hypoglycemia use the acronym: JUICE

J- Juice (such as orange or apple to increase blood sugar)

U- Unconscious patient will need IV of dextrose

I- Institute seizure precautions

C- Continue to monitor level of consciousness (LOC) and speech

E- Emergency equipment should be available (such as oral airway and suction)

Diabetes Insipidus: Signs and Symptoms

Diabetes Insipidus is a deficiency of anti-diuretic hormone (ADH) resulting in excessive water loss. Therefore, to remember the signs and symptoms of Diabetes Insipidus use the word, "WATER"

W- Water loss

A- ADH will be decreased

T- Turgor of skin will be poor

E- Excessive thirst (polydipsia) and excessive urine (polyuria)

R- Respirations will be normal

Treatment of Diabetes Insipidus

To remember the treatment of Diabetes Insipidus, use the word, "HYPOTONIC" since hypotonic fluids are used to treat the condition.

H- Hypotonic fluids (as ordered)
Y- Yes, monitor LOC
P- Pitressin (as ordered)
O- Oral hygiene and skin care
T- Thiazide diuretics (as ordered)
O- Obtain vital signs hourly
N- Na needs to be monitored
I- Iced fluids should be encouraged
C- Cerebral functioning should be monitored

Thyroid Storm: Precipitating Factors

Thyroid storm is a life threatening condition. To remember the precipitating factors that cause a thyroid storm, use one of the words from the condition: "STORM".

S- Stroke
T- Thyroid storm
O- Or inadequate treatment of hyperthyroidism
R- Results from an infection
M- Myocardial infarction or other heart failure

Symptoms of Thyroid Storm

One of the primary symptoms of thyroid storm is high fever (or febrile). Therefore, to remember the signs and symptoms of thyroid storm use the word: "FEBRILE".

> F- Febrile (fever usually between 100-105)
> E- Extreme agitation
> B- Blood pressure will be high (unless patient is in shock, then it will be low)
> R- Restlessness
> I- Increased respiratory rate
> L- LOC may be decreased
> E- Elevated T4

Chapter 2-

Muskoskeletal and

Nervous System

Preventing Bone Loss

Since Osteoporosis can be prevented with calcium, use the word: CALCIUM to prevent bone loss.

C- Calcium and vitamin D supplements

A- A weight training program

L- Light walking

C- Calcitonin

I- Implement a teaching program that includes a diet rich in calcium

U- Ultrasound used to screen for low bone density

M- Menopausal women may need hormone
    replacement therapy

Signs and Symptoms of Bells Palsy

Since Bell's palsy is a condition of the facial nerve, to remember the signs and symptoms of Bells palsy, use the word: FACIAL NERVE

    F- Facial paralysis on one side of face
    A- A dry eye on the affected side
    C- Closing of mouth difficult
    I- Increased sensitivity to sounds
    A- Affected side may have tearing
    L- Less saliva leading to dry mouth

Encephalitis

Since one of the conditions of encephalitis is a fever, to remember the symptoms of encephalitis use the word: FEVER

F- Fever and severe headache are the key
    symptoms
E- Energy loss
V- Very restless
E- Even death can occur in severe cases if
    untreated
R- Rigid, stiff neck and back

Signs and Symptoms of Impetigo

Since one of the conditions of Impetigo is a sore, use the
word "SORES " to remember the signs and symptoms
of Impetigo.

S- Sores on the skin
O- Oozing fluid from sore
R- Red small spots that change to blisters
E- Eventually breaking open of blisters
S- Sores that increase in size and number

Signs and Symptoms of ALS

To remember the signs and symptoms of Amyotrophic
lateral sclerosis (ALS) use the words: MUSCLE

M- Muscle cramps
U- Unable or difficult to lift or climb stairs

S- Slurring of speech (dysphasia) and trouble swallowing (dysphagia)

C- Cramps in muscles

L- Loss of weight

E- Eventual head drop due to weak spinal and neck muscles

Treatment of ALS

Since it is difficult to reverse the progressive disease of ALS, you can use the word, REVERSE, to remember the treatments of ALS.

R- Rilutek (is used to slow progression of disease)

E- Exercises that strengthen muscles

V- Ventilation device may be needed to assist breathing

E- Electromyogram

R- ROM exercises

S- Speech therapy (to decrease the loss of speech from disease)

E- Emotional support

Treatments of Epilepsy

To remember the treatments for seizures use the word:
ANTI-EPILEPTIC

> A- AED –Anti-Epileptic Drugs
> N- Neurontin
> T- Topiramante
> I- Including MRI
> -
> E- Epilepsy surgery
> P- Phenytoin
> I- Includes blood tests of electrolytes
> L- Levetiracetam
> E- EEG test
> P- PHT
> T- Temporal lobe resection
> I- Includes PET test
> C- Carbamazepine

Rheumatic Fever Signs and Symptoms

Since one of the main symptoms of rheumatic fever is pain in the joints, use the word, JOINTS to remember the signs and symptoms.

J- Joints are painful
O- Over a long period it can damage the heart
I- Infection may be too mild to be recognized
N- Nervous system can be affected leading to
  chorea
T- Throat that is sore
S- Swollen joints

Chapter 3- Cardiac & Renal System

Signs and Symptoms of Hypertensive Crisis

To remember the signs and symptoms of hypertensive crisis think of the word associated with blood pressure: "DIASTOLIC"

D- Dizziness
I- Increase in Heart Rate
A- A headache
S- Stroke
T- Tissue Swelling
O- Optical Disturbances
L- Level of consciousness (LOC) will change
I- Increase in diastolic BP (Greater than 130 mm/hg)
C- Changes in Pupillary Reflexes

Treatment of Hypertensive Crisis

Treatment of Hypertensive Crisis think of the word, DILATE

> D- Dilate Blood Vessels
> I- I/O monitored
> L- LOC monitored
> A-A review of BUN and Creatine
> T- Teach patient about foods high in sodium
> E- ECG monitored continuously

Signs and Symptoms of Cardiac Tamponade

To remember the signs and symptoms of Cardiac Tamponade, think of the word that rhymes with tamponade like, LEMONADE

> L- Liquid (or specifically fluid) in pericardial
>   space
> E- Elevated venous pressure with inspiration
> M- Muffled heart sounds
> O- Observe cool, pale skin
> N- Narrowed pulse pressure
> A- Anxiety, confusion
> D- Distended Jugular Veins
> E- ECG reveals widespread compression of heart

Signs and symptoms of Aortic Dissection

Aortic dissection is a tear in the aortic wall. Therefore to remember the signs and symptoms of aortic dissection use a word associated with the condition: "TEARING"

> T- Tearing pain in chest or abdomen
> E- Enlarged ascending aorta
> A- Anxiety and paleness
> R- Anxiety
> I- Race and gender is a factor as it is most common in black males
> N- Neurological changes such as lightheadedness
> G- Gas exchange is poor (due to compromised blood flow)

Causes of Renal Disease

To remember the causes of renal disease use the word: "KIDNEY"

> K- Kidney stones
> I- Increase in blood pressure, i.e., high blood pressure
> D- Diabetes (from the high blood sugar)
> N- Narrowed or blocked renal artery
> E- Enlarged prostate gland

Y- Yes, some pain meds like acetaminophen and ibuprofen

Signs and Symptoms of renal failure

To remember the signs and symptoms of renal failure use the word: "TIRED"

T- Tired or sleepy (Lethargic)
I- Irritation of stomach, i.e. nausea
R- Real trouble with sleeping
E- Edema
D- Don't feel hungry

Treatment of Chronic Renal Failure

To remember the treatments of chronic renal failure use the word: "NITROGEN"

N- Nitrogen test done, i.e. blood urea nitrogen (BUN)
I- Inhibitors such as ACE inhibitors
T- Tests of creatine
R- Restrict use of tobacco and alcohol
O- Output and Input monitored
G- Give diuretics to decrease fluid buildup
E- Exercise to help control diabetes and high blood pressure
N- Need for dialysis if renal failure is severe

Signs and Symptoms of Deep Vein Thrombosis

Deep vein thrombosis (DVT) is a blood clot in a usually in the legs. To remember the signs and symptoms of DVT use the word: CLOT

> C- Clot in deep vein
> L- Leg may ache and have swelling
> O- Overly sensitive to touch
> T- Thigh may ache

Foods High in Sodium

Patients who have cardiovascular disease or hypertension, must limit sodium intake. Therefore, to remember foods that are high in sodium use the word: CAMPBELL, as in the soup company.

C- Canned soup
A- A hot dog
M- Mixes that are instant mixes
P- Pickles
B- Bacon
E- Every type of processed food
L- Lunch meat
L- Like any type of cheese

Causes of High Cholesterol

To remember the causes of high cholesterol use the word: WEIGHT

W- Weight, being overweight can cause raise LDL and triglycerides

E- Exercise: lack of exercise

I- Inherited

G- Goods that are packaged, like cookies, and chips

H- HDL is the bad cholesterol

T- Thyroid that is low, like hypothyroidism

Uremia: Causes and Treatment

Since a diet low in potassium and protein are recommended for uremia patients, use the words "A DIET" to remember the causes and treatment of Uremia.

A- Acute Renal Failure (ACF) can be an etiology

D- Diet low in potassium and protein

I- Increased fatigue, especially in late stages

E- Elevated BUN and creatine

T- Treatment may consist of dialysis

Aortic Stenosis: Signs and Symptoms

Aortic Stenosis can occur from a narrowing of a valve. To remember the signs and symptoms of aortic stenosis use the word: "AORTIC"

A- Angina
O- Overly tired
R- Really tired and short of breath (SOB)
T- Tachycardia
I- Increase in dizziness (syncope)
C- Chance of fainting

Treatment for Aortic Stenosis

To remember some of the different types of treatments for aortic stenosis use the word associated with the disease: "BYPASS"

B- Balloon Valvuloplasty
Y- Yes, if a valve is replaced, patient may be on coumadin or heparin for life
P- Prevention of heart burn and heart failure
A- Aspirin
S- Surgery to replace aortic valve

S- Surgery consisting of a coronary artery bypass
   graft

Acute Renal Failure Signs and Symptoms

Acute renal failure usually resluts in low urine output..
One of the primary signs of acute renal failure is
oliguria (low urine). Therefore, to remember the signs
and symptoms of renal failure use the words, "LOW
URINE.

L- LOC decreased
O- Oliguria
W- Will have deep rapid respirations

U- Urea will be high (as seen in a high BUN)
R- Restlessness
I- Increased heart rate
N- Nausea
E- Elevated sodium

Treatment of Acute Renal Failure

To remember the treatment of Acute Renal Failure, use
the word: "DIALYSIS".

D- Dialysis (also Dopamine can be used here for D)

I- If hypertensive administer vasodilators (as ordered)

A- Antihypertensive (as ordered)

L- Lasix

Y- Yes, you will need to compare daily weights

S- Skin care to prevent skin breakdown

I- I/O monitored

S- Sodium and other electrolytes should be monitored

Signs and Symptoms of Hypovolemic Shock

Three types of shock are hypovolemic, cardiogenic, and anaphylactic. Since one of the causes of shock is "BLOOD LOSS" use it to remember the signs and symptoms of hypovolemic shock.

B- Blood pressure is normal

L- Lips cyanotic

O- Oxygen low in blood

O- Overactive heart rate (> 140 beats per min)

D- Delayed capillary refill

L- Lungs usually clear

O- Overactive respirations

S- Skin cool and clammy

S- Shallow rapid respirations

Signs and Symptoms of Cardiogenic Shock

Since one of the causes of cardiogenic shock is a myocardial infarction, use the word "HEART" to remember the S/S of this condition.

H- High respiratory rate (> 20)
E- Extension of MI will affect some of the signs and symptoms
A- Agitation
R- Restlessness
T- Tachycardia

Patient Management of Carotid Endarterectomy

To remember the patient management of a Carotid Endarterectomy think of the word, "REFLEX"

R- Reflex (gag) must be present before removing patient from NPO status

E- Elevate HOB 30 degrees

F- Formation of hematoma at incision site should be monitored

L- Lower HOB (if patient becomes hypotensive)

E- ECG must be monitored for possible dysrhythmias

X- X as in the roman numeral for 10 (the 10th cranial nerve, the vagus nerve may be affected)

Treatment for Patient on Dialysis

Since dialysis is used to treat Renal failure, otherwise known as "Kidney failure" use the words, "K – FAILURE" to remember the treatment of patients on dialysis.

K- Keep filters from clotting

-

F- Flatten the HOB, if patient becomes
    hypotensive

A- Aseptically clean insertion sites daily

I- Intake and output (I/O) monitored daily

L- Lower the rate of dialysis if cramping occurs
    in extremities

U- Use strict aseptic techniques during
    exchanges

R- Reduce dialysis rate if patient gets headache,
    nausea/vomiting or seizures

E- Elevate HOB (if patient develops tachypnea
    and dyspnea

Digoxin: Patient Management

To remember the patient management of patients on
Digoxin, think of the effect it has on patients which is to
make the heart beat stronger. Therefore, to remember
the patient management use the words, "STRONG
H.R." as in *strong heart rate.*

S- Serum potassium levels should be checked before administering

T- Take apical pulse for 1 minute. (If < 60 withhold and notify physician)

R- Rate of heart rate will decline when administered

O- Overdose is treated with magnesium sulfate

N- Nausea/vomiting is a side effect

G- Give cautiously in elderly patients

H- Hypokalemia is associated with increased risk for digitalis toxicity

-

R- Renal blood flow will increase when administered

Signs and Symptoms of Cardiac Tamponade

To remember the signs and symptoms of Cardiac Tamponade, use the word, "PERICARDIAL"

P- Pericardial space is filled with excess fluid

E- Echocardiogram to reveal congestion

R- Relieve cardiac compression

I- Increase in venous pressure with inspiration

C- Capillary refill less than 3 seconds

A- Anxiety

R- Rub from pericardium may be present

D- Decreased cardiac output

I- Increased Jugular Vein distention (JVD)

A- A pacemaker, chest trauma and renal failure may be risk factors

L- Level of consciousness must be assessed for changes that may indicate decreased cerebral perfusion

Signs and Symptoms and Treatment of Hypertensive Crisis

For the S/S and Treatment of Hypertensive Crisis, use the acronym: CRISIS

C- Calcium channel blockers

R- Rest to decrease myocardial oxygen demand

I- Infusion of Vasodilators may be ordered

S- Surgical intervention may be needed

I- Ischemia

S- Sympatholytics

Pretest and Post-Test of Intravenous Pyelogram

To remember the pretest and post-test of Intravenous Pyelogram (IVP), use the word: IODINE

I- Iodine or seafood allergies need to be assessed on patient before test

O- Oliguria should be checked: urine should be greater than 30ml/hr

D- Do not administer test if BUN is less than 40 mg/dl

I- Infection is possible from catheterization

N- NPO 4 to 6 hours before the test

E- Encourage fluids after the test

Treatment of Angina Pectoris

To remember the treatment of Angina pectoris use the acronym: CALCIUM

C- Calcium channel blockers

A- Administer nitroglycerine

L- Low levels of Oxygen (i.e., 02 at 2 L)

C- Cardiac catheterization in extreme cases

I- Initiate and maintain an IV line

U- Use bed rest and ECG

M- Monitor drug effects on HR and BP

Signs and Symptoms of Myocardial Infarction

To remember the signs and symptoms of myocardial infarction (MI) think of the word: MYOCARDIAL

> M- Murmur and or cardiac rubs may be present
> Y- Yes, there will be Shortness of breath (SOB)
> O- Oxygen saturation will be low
> C- CK-MB cardiac enzymes are present 16-24 hours after MI
> A- Anxious, pale
> R- Respiratory assessment will reveal clear lungs
> D- Diaphoresis and Distended jugular veins
> I- Iso-enzymes are elevated (CK-MB, AST, LDH) are indicative of MI
> A- AST cardiac enzymes are present 24-48 hours after MI
> L- LDH cardiac enzymes are present 48-72 hours after MI

Treatment of Myocardial Infarction

To remember treatments for myocardial infarction (MI) think of the word: HEART

> H- Heparin

E- ECG monitoring to evaluate signs of ischemia, or infarction

A- Antihypertensives

R- Rest in bed

T- Thrombolytic therapy

Signs and Symptoms of Congestive Heart Failure (CHF)

The side of the heart failure will dictate some differences in signs and symptoms of heart failure. However, to remember the signs and symptoms of congestive heart failure (CHF), use the acronym below: LOW CARDIAC OUT

L- Low cardiac output is cause of CHF

O- Orthopnea

W- White, pale skin

C- Cardiomegaly

A- Ascites

R- Right Upper quadrant pain (if right-sided failure)

D- Dependant edema

I- Increased heart rate

A- Anorexia

C- Crackles

Treatment of Congestive Heart Failure (CHF)

To remember the treatment of congestive heart failure (CHF) use the word: LANOXIN

> L- Lanoxin / Lasix
> A- Apical pulse - taken for 1 minute before
>   giving (Lanoxin); hold if < 60 heart rate
> N- NPO may be ordered in acute phase
> O- Oxygen at 2-4 L/min
> X- X-ray (of chest may reveal enlarged heart)
> I- IV lines for emergency drugs
> N- Nitroglycerine (NTG) may be ordered

Signs and Symptoms & Treatment of Pulmonary Edema

Since Pulmonary Edema is the accumulation of fluid in the lung, use the phrase "FLUID in the LUNGS" to remember some of the signs and symptoms and treatment of pulmonary edema.

> S/S:
> F- Fluid in the lungs
> L- Life threatening situation

U- Usually shortness of breath (SOB)
I- Impaired gas exchange
D- Discomfort in the chest

Treatment:

L- Low dose morphine may be ordered to
decrease anxiety
U- Urine output and electrolytes are monitored
N- NPO
G- Give diuretics to decrease fluid on lungs

Signs and Symptoms of Pericarditis

Since Pericarditis involves an infection of the
pericardium, use the word "INFECTIONS " to
remember the signs and symptoms of pericarditis

I- Infections can be a risk factor to pericarditis
N- Neoplasms can be a risk factor to pericarditis
F- Friction rub is a symptom
E- Echocardiogram may indicate pericardial
effusion
C- Cardiac enzymes are usually normal unless a
myocardial infarction is involved
T- Tachypnea
I- Irritability
O- Often difficult breathing
N- Normally patient will have increased HR and
temperature

S- Severe, sharp pain

Signs and Symptoms of Cardiomyopathy

To remember the signs and symptoms of cardiomyopathy use the word: MYOPATH

> M- Murmurs
> Y- Yes, there can be either hypertension or hypotension depending on the etiology
> O- Oxygen at 2-4 L/min
> P- Pulmonary crackles
> A- A dry cough
> T- Tachycardia
> H- Heart failure

Treatment of Endocarditis

Endocarditis is the inflammation of the endocardium. It usually is caused by viral, fungal, or bacteria. Therefore, to remember the treatment for endocarditis use a word from one the agents that causes endocarditis: BACTERIA

> B- Bedrest
> A- Antibiotic therapy

C- Central venous pressure (CVP) monitored
T- Temperature monitored as fever is the most
   common early manifestation
E- ECG every 4 hours
R- Review BUN and Creatine levels
I- Initiate and maintain I.V. line
A- A diuretic

Causes of High Central Venous Pressure (CVP)

To remember the causes of high CVP use, OVERLOAD, while using LOWS to remember the causes of low CVP.

High CVP
O- Overload of fluids
V- Ventricular septal defect
E- Embolus (pulmonary embolus)
R- Right ventricular infarction
L- Lungs have defects: ie, COPD
O- Or retention of fluid
A- A case of pericarditis
D- Disease of tricuspid or pulmonic heart valves

Causes of Low Central Venous Pressure (CVP)

<u>Low CVP</u>
L- Low fluid volume
O- Overuse of diuretics
W- Will occur with drug use
S- Sepsis

Chapter 4- Gastrointestinal System

Gastro-esophageal Reflux Disease signs and symptoms

Since the most common GERD symptom is chronic heartburn, use the word: H-BURN to remember the signs and symptoms of this condition.

H- Heartburn

B- Bad breath; belching
U- Unusual sour taste in mouth
R- Real chance of tooth erosion
N- Nagging hoarseness

Causes of Gastro-esophageal Reflux Disease (GERD)

To remember the causes and conditions that irritate Gastro-esophageal Reflux Disease (GERD) use the word: BROWNIES

> B- Being overweight
> R- Really large portions of food
> O- Onions
> W- Wearing tight fitting clothing or belts
> N- Nighttime eating before bedtime
> I- Ingesting certain beverages like citrus juices, alcohol, caffeinated and carbonated drinks
> E- Eating chocolate, high fat or spicy foods
> S- Smoking

Treatments for GERD

To remember the treatments for GERD, use the word: MEDITATION

C- Crohn's disease
E- Eating to few folate rich foods (such as vegetables or overcooking vegetables)
L- Loss of blood
L- Little iron in diet
S- Sickle Cell

Risk factors of Gastric Cancer

Gastric cancer can sometimes run in the family. Therefore, to remember the conditions that can increase the risk of gastric cancer use the word: FAMILY

F- Family history of gastric cancer
A- A diet high in salted, smoked or preserved foods
M- Male gender
I- Incidence of gastric polyps
L- Low fruits and vegetables in diet
Y- Yes, it occurs more in advanced age

Signs and Symptoms of Gastric Cancer

One of the common symptoms of gastric cancer is heartburn. Therefore, to remember the signs and symptoms of gastric cancer use the word: HEARTBURN.

> H- Heartburn
> E- Enlarged lymph nodes
> A- Anemia / A loss of appetite
> R- Results in weight loss
> T- Tarry, black stools
> B- Bloated feeling after eating
> U- Upper or middle part of abdomen has discomfort
> R- Results in vomiting
> N- Nausea

Gastric cancer is diagnosed with an upper GI.

Signs and Symptoms of Cholecystitis

Cholecystitis is inflammation of the gallbladder, usually caused by gallstones. Therefore, to remember the signs and symptoms of Cholecystitis use the word:

S- Shoulder blade (on right side) or back pain

T- Tenderness in the right abdomen

O- Occurs more frequently in females (than males) / Obesity increases incidence

N- Nausea or vomiting

E- Edema of the gallbladder leading to pain

S- Sometimes pain for more than 6 hours after meals

Treatment of Cholecystitis

To remember the treatment for Cholecystitis use one of the words associated with gallbladder: BILE

B- Begin low fat diet after surgery

I- Immediate cholecystectomy in severe cases

L- Lab studies to find no evidence of obstruction (in mild cases)

E- Emesis can be treated with antiemetics

Signs and Symptoms of Diverticulosis

Since diverticulosis has outward pouches in the colon, use the word "OUTWARD" to remember the signs and symptoms of diverticulosis.

O- Occasional cramping
U- Usually identified on CT scan
T- Temperature will be normal
W- Will not have symptoms (for most patients)
A- Abdominal pain
R- Regular exercise, high fiber diet and 8 glasses of water will decrease diverticulosis
D- Diarrhea

Signs and Symptoms of Irritable Bowel Syndrome

Irritable bowel syndrome (IBS) contains the word irritable. Therefore, to remember the signs and symptoms of IBS use the word: IRRITABLE

I- Insomnia

R- Results in having more than 3 bowel
movements a day

R- Really tired

I- Intestines may have feeling of gas

T- Taste of food may be unpleasant

A- Anxiety or depression

B- Bowel movements differ in size or consistency

L- Lower back pain

E- Emptying of bladder difficult

Signs and Symptoms of Acute Peritonitis

Acute peritonitis is the inflammation of the peritoneal
cavity. To remember the signs and symptoms use the
words from one of the symptoms: "KNEES FLEXED"

K- Knees flexed

N- Normal to decreased mentation

E- Elevated heart rate

E- Elevated

S- Severe pain

F- Flushed pale skin

L- Low electrolyte levels

E- Elevated WBC count

X- X-rays detect air in the abdomen

E- Elevated BUN and creatine

D- Distended abdomen with rebound tenderness

Upper GI Bleeding Signs and Symptoms

Upper Gastrointestinal (GI) bleeding is bleeding sometimes caused by a peptic ulcer. Therefore, to remember the signs and symptoms of upper GI bleeding use the word, PEPTIC.

> P- Pain at the peptic ulcer site
> E- Emesis
> P- Pain will be absent if it is from esophageal varices
> T- Thready weak pulse
> I- Irritated or apprehensive
> C- Cool clammy skin is possible

Treatment of Esophageal Varices

To remember the treatment of Esophageal Varices think of the word associated with the condition: "VARICES"

V- Vasopressin (as ordered)
A- Anticipate balloon tamponade
R- Restrain patient (as ordered)
I- Infiltration of vasopressin during IV may
   cause necrosis
C- Continuously monitor vital signs
E- Endoscopic sclerotherapy
S- Secure all tubes to prevent dislodgement and
excessive movement that can cause gastric irritation

Precautions for patients on Enteric feedings

Precautions for patients on enteric feedings: To remember
the reasons to consult a physician for a patient who in on
enteric feedings, think of the word associated with not
feeding someone, namely, "DON'T FEED".

D- Dehydration
O- Output of gastric residual > 50 % of delivery
   rate
N- No bowel sounds
T- Tube displacement

F- Feeding tube has mucosal damage
E- Elevated serum glucose
E- Evidence of possible aspiration
D- Diarrhea that is uncontrolled

Barium Enema Preparation

ENEMA is a good word association for pretest patient management for patients who are undergoing a Barium Enema

> E- Ensure Hydration
> N- NPO after midnight
> E- Evacuation of Barium should occur within 24-72 hours
> M- Motility (of the intestines is decreased with narcotics, so withhold them)
> A- Administer Laxatives after the test

Signs and Symptoms of Crohn' s Disease

To remember the s/s of Crohn's Disease use the acronym: "ULCERATIONS".

> U- Ulcerations of the intestinal mucosa
> L- Loss of weight
> C- Chronic diarrhea with blood
> E- Elevated Temperature
> R- Right quadrant pain
> A- Abdominal cramps after meals

T- Test positive for fecal fat
I- Inflammatory disease of small intestine
O- Occult blood in feces
N- Nausea
S- Slowly progressive with exacerbations and
   remissions

Treatment of Crohn' s Disease

A- Avoid laxatives
V- Vitamins and minerals
O- Observe for signs of rectal hemorrhage
I- IV therapy: heparin lock
D- Demerol

L- Lab studies
A- A potassium supplement
X- eXercise regularly
A- Alternate rest periods with activity
T- TPN
I- Identify ways to reduce stress
V- Vital signs monitored
E- Environment that's quiet
S- Stop smoking

Assessment Findings and Treatment

Aplastic Anemia

To remember the treatment and assessment findings of aplastic anemia think of one of the words that is associated with it, "MARROW".

> M- Marrow (bone marrow) transplant
> A- Aspiration of bone marrow to diagnose the condition
> R- RBC's will be low
> R- Requires cortisone to stop autoimmune process
> O- Occurs as congenital or acquired
> W- WBC's will be low

Chapter 5-

Respiratory System

Signs and Symptoms of Tuberculosis (TB)

Since one the common signs and symptoms of Tuberculosis is loose secretions (mucus) you should use the word LOOSE to remember the signs and symptoms of Tuberculosis.

L- Lymph nodes swollen
O- Ongoing cough
O- Occasionally chest pain or SOB
S- Sputum
E – Elevated heart rate: Tachycardia

Treatment of Tuberculosis

When you think of the treatment for tuberculosis, think of this: If you are RIPE, you will cough from Tuberculosis. Therefore, to remember the treatments of tuberculosis use the word: RIPE

R- Rifampin
I- Isoniazid
P- Pyrazinamide
E- Ethambutol

Signs and Symptoms of Anaphylactic Shock

Anaphylactic shock is a very serious condition of the respiratory system where the patient has difficulty in breathing. Therefore, to remember the S/S of anaphylactic shock use the phrase, "CAN'T BREATH.

C- Chest tightness
A- Anxiety
N- Neuro will be low (may be unresponsive)
T- Tachycardia

B- Breathing will be difficult (i.e. SOB)
R- Restlessness
E- Epinephrine (as ordered)
A- Aminophylline (as ordered)
T- Tube (i.e. intubations)
H- Have to give oxygen

Signs and Symptoms of Pulmonary Emboli

To remember the signs and symptoms of Pulmonary Emboli, use the word phrase: BLOOD CLOT

> B- Blood pressure is increased
> L-LOC is altered in severe cases
> O- Occurrence of patechiae may occur
> O- Oxygen: administer oxygen
> D- Deep vein thrombosis (DVT) may occur in severe cases
>
> C- Crackles
> L-Long bone fracture may cause emboli
> O- Overly colorful skin (i.e., petechiae
> T – Tachypnea and tachycardia many occur

Signs and Symptoms of Acute Respiratory Distress Syndrome

To remember the signs and symptoms of Acute Respiratory Distress Syndrome (ARDS) use the word: DISTRESS

> D- Dyspnea
> I- Increased heart rate due to hypoxemia
> S- Signs of cyanosis in late stages

T- Tachypnea

R- Restlessness

E- ECG may be needed for signs of myocardial
   ischemia

S- Sensations will be decreased

S- Status of BP may be increased or decreased

Signs and Symptoms of Pneumonia

To remember the signs and symptoms of pneumonia
use the acronym: PURULENT

P- Purulent or rust colored sputum

U- Upper airway and lower airways may be
   obstructed

R- Respiratory rate above 24 per min

U- Unusually wet skin (ie: Diaphoresis)

L- Level of consciousness (LOC) may be altered

E- Electrolyte imbalance may reveal acidosis

N- Nutrition may be altered resulting in less
   than body requirements

T- Tachycardia and temperature will be high

Chapter 6-
Pediatrics

Spina Bifida Treatment

Spina Bifica is a condition of a spine disorder.
Therefore, to remember the signs and symptoms and
treatment of spina bifida use the words: SPINE
DISORDER

S- Seizure disorders is some cases
P- Problems with breathing during sleep
I- In mild cases of spina bifida there may be no
  signs
N- Nerves and tissues are exposed from spinal
  cord in severe cases
E- Edema on the child's spine

D- Difficulty swallowing and choking
I- Incontinence
S- Strabismus

O- Often results in scoliosis, kyphosis, or both.
R- Recommended that child receives stool
softener
D- Drainage tube if child has hydrocephalus
E- Examinations such as amniocentesis and
ultrasound to test for spina bifida
R- Renal ultrasound to test for damage of the
kidneys

Symptoms of Reye's syndrome

Since Reyes syndrome can happen rapidly, use the word RAPID to remember the signs and symptoms of Reye's syndrome.

R- Rapid development of symptoms
A- Aggressive behavior
P- Positioning of body abnormal
I- inability to identify whereabouts or family
members or to answer simple questions
D- Deep breathing

Treatment of Reye' s syndrome

To remember the treatments of Reye's syndrome use the word: BRAIN

B- Brain swelling is prevented by osmotic
   diuretics
R- Respirator used if difficulty in breathing
A- A Foley catheter may be needed
I- I/O monitored
N- NPO

Signs and Symptoms of Klinefelter Syndrome

Since signs and symptoms of Klinefelter syndrome do
not usually appear until puberty, use the word,
PUBERTY to remember the signs and symptoms.

P- Pelvis area will be wide (i.e. wide hips)
U- Unusually long legs and narrow shoulders
B- Be taller than other males in their family
E- Enlarged breasts (gynecomastia)
R- Reduced verbal skills and social skills /
   Retardation in some cases
T- Testosterone levels will be low (men may be
   infertile)
Y- Y chromosomes will be less than X
   chromosome

Diagnosing Klinefelter Syndrome

Since a chromosome <u>test</u> is used diagnose klinefelter syndrome use the word <u>TEST</u> to remember the medical exams and treatments of klinefelter syndrome.

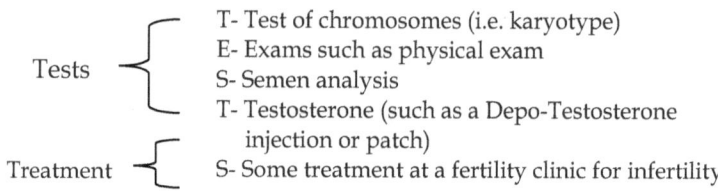

Tests
- T- Test of chromosomes (i.e. karyotype)
- E- Exams such as physical exam
- S- Semen analysis
- T- Testosterone (such as a Depo-Testosterone injection or patch)

Treatment
- S- Some treatment at a fertility clinic for infertility

Assessment Findings for Failure to Thrive (FTT)

To remember the assessment findings and interventions for a child who has failure to thrive (FTT), use a word from one of the symptoms: "RUMINATION".

R- Rumination

U- Urge the parents to establish and maintain a structured routine

M- Mental age and chronological age may not be the same

I- Inadequate feeding techniques should be corrected

N- Need to rule out physiologic causes

A- Act as a role model for parents

T- Talking or smiling may be absent

I- Infants are commonly the ones affected

O- Observe for sleep disturbances as growth hormone is released during sleep

N- Note the child's history for insufficient stimulation

Signs and Symptoms of Down's Syndrome

Since Down's syndrome is a condition affiliated with trisomy 21, to remember the signs and symptoms of this condition use the word, "TRISOMY".

T- Total of 47 chromosomes

R- Risk of congenital heart defects

I- Immune system may be weak

S- Small head with slow brain growth

O- Oral cavity small leading to protruding tongue

M- Moderate retardation

Y- You will notice small skin folds on the inner corner of the eyes

Assessment Findings of Aspirin Poisoning

To remember some of the assessment findings from aspirin poisoning, use a word form one of the symptoms: "TINNITUS".

T- Tinnitus

I- Increased respiratory rate

N- Normal dose is 1grain per year of age (up to age 10)

N- Note decrease in blood glucose levels

I- Irritation of GI tract

T- Two to four hours is the it takes aspirin to reach its peak effect

U- Upset GI system

S- Supplements of calcium and potassium (as ordered)

Treatment of Acetaminophen Poisoning

To remember the treatment for acetaminophen poisoning think of the word that is one of the interventions: "EMESIS"

> E- Emesis should be induced
> M- Maintain a patent airway
> E- Evaluate for liver damage 24-36 hours after overdose
> S- Serum plasma levels greater than 200 mcg/ml will lead to hepatotoxicity
>
> I-Ipecac syrup (to induce vomiting)
> S- Symptoms such as nausea/vomiting and diarrhea should be assessed

To remember the assessment findings of a child with lead poisoning think of one of the words from the condition, "LEAD".

> L- Lead lines will be seen along
> E- Evaluate for bone pain
> A- Assess for anemia
> D- Determine blood lead levels via an erythrocyte protoporphyrin test

Findings and Interventions of Rocky Mountain Spotted Fever

To remember some of the key features and interventions of Rocky Mountain spotted fever, think of the first word from the condition, "ROCKY"

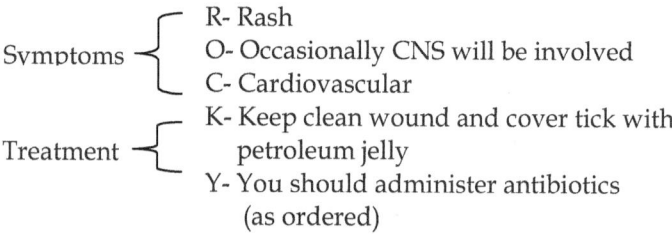

Symptoms
- R- Rash
- O- Occasionally CNS will be involved
- C- Cardiovascular

Treatment
- K- Keep clean wound and cover tick with petroleum jelly
- Y- You should administer antibiotics (as ordered)

Treatment of Anemia in Children

To remember the treatment of anemia in children, think of the word from the condition, "ANEMIA"

A- Assess for hepatomegaly

N- Note growth retardation and gum
 hypertrophy

E- Eliminate the cause of anemia

M- Maintain normal body temperature

I- Iron rich foods, such as dark leafy vegetables
 and whole grains

A- Administer iron before meals with juice
 (Rationale: Iron is best absorbed in an
 acidic environment)

Signs and Symptoms of Hemophilia

To remember the signs and symptoms of Hemophilia,
think of a word from one of the symptoms,
"BLEEDIMG".

B- Bleeding easily after circumcision,
 immunizations

L- Limited joint mobility

E- Elevated PTT

E- Excessive bruises without petechiae

D- Degeneration of joint (from hemarthrases)

I- Increased risk of HIV from blood transfusions

N- Note swelling, or pain of joints

G- Genetic counseling should be offered to
 affected parents

Signs and Symptoms and Treatment of Meningitis

To remember some of the signs and symptoms and treatment of meningitis think of one of the symptoms, "KERNIGS SIGN".

Signs and Symptoms
- K- Kernigs sign
- E- Ear drainage
- R- Rash
- N- Notice Brudzinski's sign
- I- Intracranial pressure (ICP) increased
- G- Glucose in cerebral spinal fluid (CSF)
- S- Seizures may occur

Treatment
- S- Seizure precautions
- I- Isolate child after antibiotic therapy starts
- G- Gently move child
- N- Neuro status monitored frequently

Chapter 7- OB/GYN

Risk Factors of Gestational Diabetes

To remember the risk factors for patients with gestational diabetes use the word:

> O- Older than 35 years of age
> L- Low weight of newborn
> D- Demise of fetus in past that is unexplained
> E- Extreme weight of mother
> R- Rise in fasting glucose that is greater than 140 mg/dl

Preeclampsia: Signs and Symptoms

Since headache is one of the symptoms of Preeclampsia, to remember the signs and symptoms of preeclampsia use the word: HEADACHE

> H- Headache
> E- Elevated protein in urine
> A- Abruptio placenta

D- Dizziness

A- A low birth weight for the neonate

C- Changes in visual perception

H- High blood pressure: systolic >160mm Hg or diastolic > 110mm Hb

E- Edema

Treatment of Preeclampsia

Magnesium sulfate is used to treat preeclampsia. Therefore, to remember the treatment of preeclampsia use a shortened version of magnesium sulfate word: MAG

M- Magnesium sulfate

A- Antihypertensive meds

G- Give low-dose aspirin and electrolytes

RH Factor and the need for RhoGAM

Since Rh factor is used to determine the need for RhoGAM use the word: FACTOR

F- Fetal Doppler ultrasound

A- Amniocentesis to determine blood type and Rh factor

C- Coombs test to check for increase in Rh positive antibody levels

T- Testing should occur in first trimester

O- On a repeated basis, amniocentesis is to monitor how fetus is affected by sensitization

R- Rh sensitization is necessary to ensure fetus can be monitored and treated

Signs and Symptoms of Endometriosis

Since the patient can have pain during ovulation, think of the word OVULATE to remember the signs and symptoms and treatment of endometriosis.

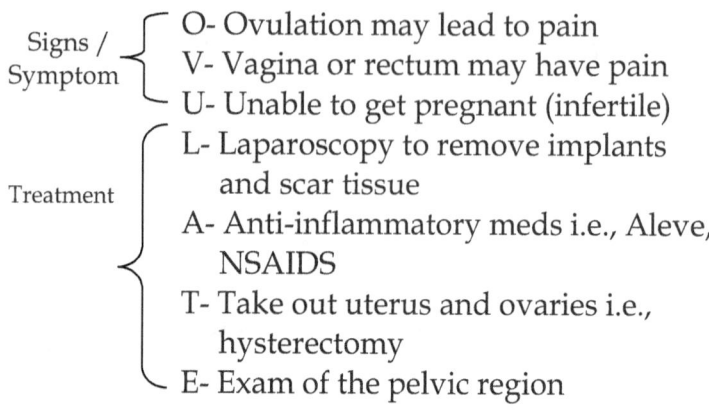

Signs /
Symptom
- O- Ovulation may lead to pain
- V- Vagina or rectum may have pain
- U- Unable to get pregnant (infertile)

Treatment
- L- Laparoscopy to remove implants and scar tissue
- A- Anti-inflammatory meds i.e., Aleve, NSAIDS
- T- Take out uterus and ovaries i.e., hysterectomy
- E- Exam of the pelvic region

Signs and Symptoms of Cerebral Palsy

To remember the signs and symptoms and treatment of cerebral palsy think of one of the symptoms, "SPEECH DEFICIT".

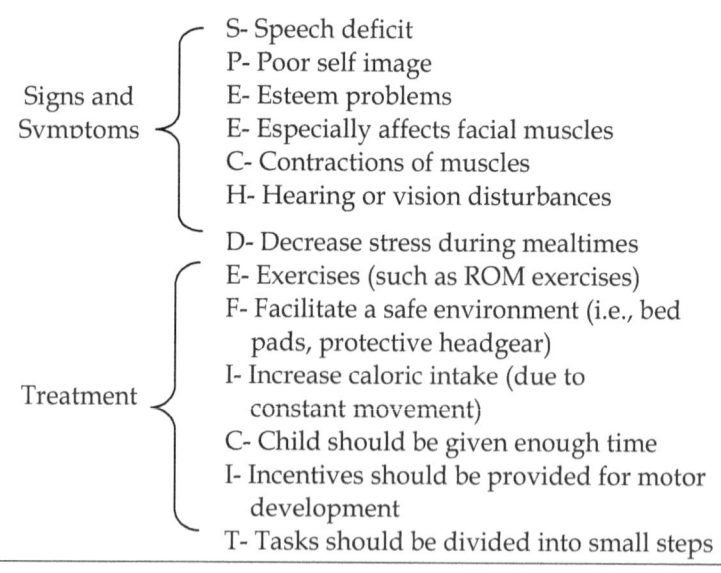

Signs and
Symptoms
- S- Speech deficit
- P- Poor self image
- E- Esteem problems
- E- Especially affects facial muscles
- C- Contractions of muscles
- H- Hearing or vision disturbances

Treatment
- D- Decrease stress during mealtimes
- E- Exercises (such as ROM exercises)
- F- Facilitate a safe environment (i.e., bed pads, protective headgear)
- I- Increase caloric intake (due to constant movement)
- C- Child should be given enough time
- I- Incentives should be provided for motor development
- T- Tasks should be divided into small steps

Signs and Symptoms of Hydrocephalus

To remember the signs and symptoms of hydrocephalus (before closure of cranial sutures) think of the words, "BIG HEAD".

> B- Big head
> I- Irritability
> G- Going to have decreased attention span
> -
> H- High pitched cry
> E- Extended bulging fontanels
> A- A widening of suture lines
> D- Distended scalp veins

Treatment for Hydrocephalus

To remember the treatment for hydrocephalus, think of a word from one of the treatment interventions: "SHUNT".

> S- Shunt inserted
> H- Head of bed (HOB) elevated
> U- Urinary incontinence may occur in children (if shunt fails or malfunctions)
> N- Need to observe for shunt blockage as noted with signs of increased ICP.
> T- Take care of the head with proper skin care

Chapter 8-

Pharmacology

Nursing

Side Effects and PT Teaching of Zocor

To remember some of the teaching methods and side effects of this medication think of the words: NO GRAPEFRUIT.

Patient
Teaching
{ N- No grapefruit or grapefruit juice
while taking Zocor
O- Orally taken

Side
Effects
{ G- Gastric pain
R- Rhabdomyolysis (is a possible side effect)
A- A serious allergic reaction is unlikely but may occur
P- Persistent nausea
E- Eyes and skin may become yellow
F- Fatigue

R- Rash
U- Urine may be dark
I- Itching
T- Trouble breathing

Side Effects of Zoloft

Zoloft is an antidepressant. To remember the side effects of this medication think of the words, DRY MOUTH

D- Dry mouth
R- Really sweaty
Y- Yellow eyes and skin

M- May have black stools
O- Oral mucosa may have bleeding
U- Upset stomach
T- Trouble sleeping
H- Have trouble staying awake (i.e., sleepy)

Side Effects of Buspar

Buspar is an anti-anxiety. Since it is used to relieve anxiety and stress, use the word RELAX to remember some of its side effects and precautions.

R- Restlessness
E- Expression on face may be mask-like
L- Lightheadedness
A- A blurry vision
X- X-tra care when pregnant as the medicine can be passed with breast milk

Side Effects of Cipro

Cipro is an antibiotic. To remember the precautions and side effects of this medication think of one of its potential side effects: DARK URINE

D- Dark Urine

A- A yellowing of eyes or skin (jaundice)

R- Rare thoughts of suicide

K- Knee or joint pain or swelling

U- Unusual tiredness

R- Rise in body temperature (febrile)

I- Irregular heartbeat

N- Need to drink plenty of fluids

E- Easy bruising

Etiologies of Blood Clots

Warfarin (Coumadin) is used to prevent and treat harmful blood clots Warfarin is an anticoagulant. To remember some possible etiologies for blood clots use the word: HEART.

H- Heart valve replacement

E- Events of irregular heart rhythm

A- Atrial fibrillation

R- Recent heart attack

T- Types of conditions that cause stagnant blood to collect

Teaching patients about Coumadin

Precautions and teaching methods for patients on Coumadin can be remembered by using the word: "PLAY"

P- Prothrombin time (PT) needs to be monitored

L- Liver, broccoli, and other green leafy vegetables contain vitamin K and therefore should be avoided

A- Avoid cranberry juice because it can increase effects of coumadin

Y- Yes, patient should consult physician if they experience sudden intense pain or weakness on one side of their body

Types of Antidepressant Medications

To remember the major types of antidepressants use this phrase by using the first letter of each word: "May The Serotonin Satisfy"

M- MAO inhibitors (MAO)

T- Tricyclic antidepressants (TCA)

S- Serotonin reuptake inhibitors (SRI)

S- Serotonin and norepinephrine reuptake inhibitors

• Many of the (TCAs) cause dry mouth

- Many of the (MAO's) cause heart problems like chest pain or tachycardia

Signs and Symptoms of Conjunctivitis

Conjunctivitis is redness and swelling of the conjunctiva leading to redness and edema. Since the main cause for the spread of conjunctivitis is poor hand washing use the word SOAP to remember the signs and symptoms of conjunctivitis.

S- Swollen, red eyelids
O- Occasional drainage from eye
A- An itching or burning
P- Photophobia

Abbreviations for Administering Eye Drops

The different abbreviations for eyes are OD, OS, and OU. To remember the abbreviations for eye drops use the following scenario:

- Most people have a dominant right hand; therefore, think of OD as meaning drops in right eye.

- Then, think that fewer people are somewhat left handed; as a result, OS means to place drops in left eye.

- Lastly, OU being the only reaming abbreviation, use it to remember that it means both eyes.

Treatment of Glaucoma

Since one of the symptoms of Glaucoma is tunnel vision, think of the word car in Pilocarpine. Then, to remember the treatment of glaucoma, think of a car (from the word Pilo**car**pine) driving through a tunnel. Then, you can associate Pilo**car**pine as a medication used to treat glaucoma, which has tunnel vision as one of its symptoms.

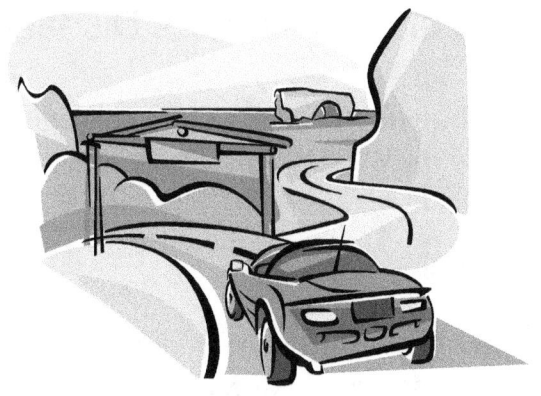

Treatment of Shingles

While having shingles will give you a rash, it will not give you black and white stripes like that of a zebra. Therefore, to remember the treatment of shingles use the word: ZEBRA

> Z- Zovirax (as ordered)
> E- Eye or face shingles may have to be treated with corticosteroids
> B- Be careful as pt. with shingles can spread chickenpox
> R- Relieve pain with narcotics or NSAIDS (as ordered)
> A- Advil

Symptoms of Parkinson' s Disease

Since one of the symptoms of Parkinson's disease (PD) is shaking, use the word SHAKING to remember the symptoms of PD.

S- Shaking
H- Hands trembling
A- Automatic and spontaneous movement decreases (bradykinesia)
K- Key symptom can be slow movement and reduced arm swing
I- Inherited (it may be inherited)
N- Nighttime problems such as <u>difficulty</u> sleeping
G- Gait will be unsteady and difficult

Side Effects of Levodopa

The drug of choice for Parkinson's disease is Levodopa. Since it is used to control motor function, think of the word, MOTOR

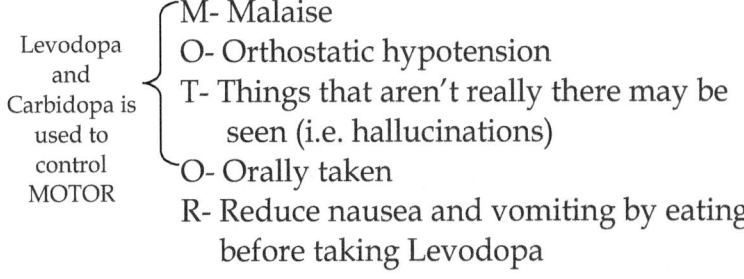

Levodopa and Carbidopa is used to control MOTOR

M- Malaise
O- Orthostatic hypotension
T- Things that aren't really there may be seen (i.e. hallucinations)
O- Orally taken
R- Reduce nausea and vomiting by eating before taking Levodopa

Signs and Symptoms of Lyme Disease

Lyme disease is the most common tick-borne illness in the United States. To remember the signs and symptoms of Lyme disease think of the word: TICKS

T- Tired, fatigued is the most common symptom
I- Inability to control muscles of the face (Bells Palsy)
C- Chills and fever
K- Knees and joints may have swelling
S- Swollen Lymph nodes

Uses of Atropine Sulfate

To remember the key features of Atropine Sulfate think of a word from the last part of Atropine, namely, "pine" and then add "TREE" to remember some of the uses of atropine sulfate.

T-Treats bradycardia
R- Rate of heart should be > 60 when thereby is working
E- Emergencies, it can be given IV push
E- Excessive doses can lead to tachycardia

Bumex: Patient Management

To remember some of the patient management for Bumex, just use the same word, "BUMEX".

B- Blood pressure and heart rate monitored
U- Used for edema, and CHF
M- More potent than Lasix |
E- Evaluate hearing and check for ototoxicity
X- eXamine for volume depletion (i.e., thirst)

Epinephrine: Side Effects

Epinephrine is a bronchodilator used to treat anaphylaxis and cardiac arrest. To remember some of the side effects and patient management of Epinephrine think of the last part of the word, namely, "NEPHRINE"

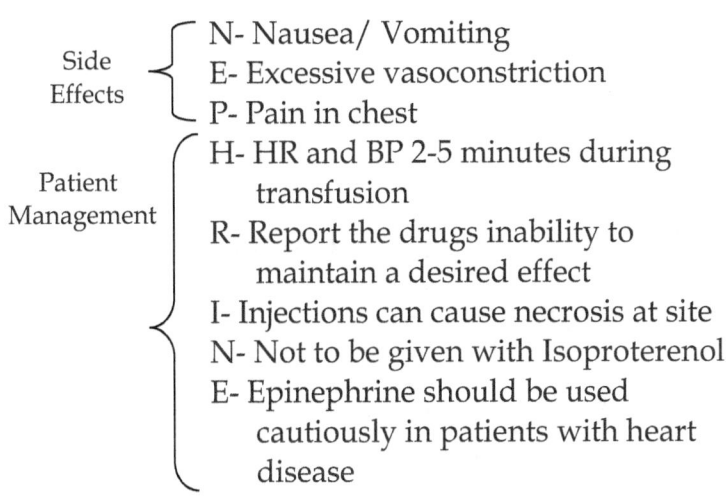

Side Effects
- N- Nausea/ Vomiting
- E- Excessive vasoconstriction
- P- Pain in chest

Patient Management
- H- HR and BP 2-5 minutes during transfusion
- R- Report the drugs inability to maintain a desired effect
- I- Injections can cause necrosis at site
- N- Not to be given with Isoproterenol
- E- Epinephrine should be used cautiously in patients with heart disease

Lasix: Side Effects

Lasix is a loop diuretic. To remember the side effects and patient management think of the type of medication Lasix is, namely, "DIURETIC"

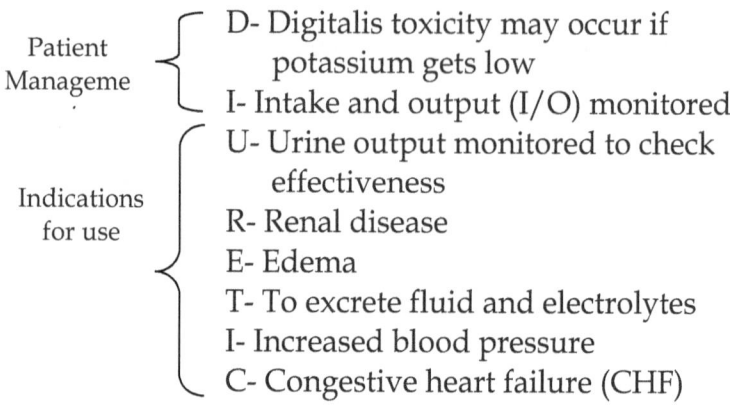

Patient Manageme.
- D- Digitalis toxicity may occur if potassium gets low
- I- Intake and output (I/O) monitored

Indications for use
- U- Urine output monitored to check effectiveness
- R- Renal disease
- E- Edema
- T- To excrete fluid and electrolytes
- I- Increased blood pressure
- C- Congestive heart failure (CHF)

Pediatric Medication Administration Procedures

To remember some of the medication administration procedures for pediatric patients, use the word, "PRE-PUBERTY"

P- Pain may be associated with punishment by the child

R- Reinforce the fact that pain is not a punishment

E- Encourage child to express feelings by providing play

-

P- Pills should be crushed for infants and young children

U- Under age 3, do not inject into dorsogluteal muscle

B- Bandage adhesive for minor pain

E- Encourage child to assist with painful procedures such as removing a bandage

R- Remember that a hospitalized child faces specialized difficulties

T- Tell the child when something will hurt

Y- You should select the needle length according to the patients muscle size

Antidepressants

To remember medicines classified as antidepressants use one of the antidepressant medicines as the acronym: "MARPLAN".

M- Marplan
A- Amitriptyline
R- Rapiflux
P- Parnate
L- Lexapro
A- Amoxapine
N- Nardil

Chapter 9- Fluid and Electrolytes

Arterial Blood Gases

5 Tips for ABG's

1. Sodium Bicarbonate: To remember HCO3 (Sodium Bicarbonate), associate it with "Buy-a-car-bonate". The typical age for consumers buying their first car is 22-26 years old (their first purchase without parents purchasing it, and for the sake of this study). So, "Buy-a-car-bonate" (or bicarbonate) is 22-26.

2. Normal blood pH is 7.35 – 7.45. Normal CO2 is 35 – 45. Notice that both have common numbers: they both have 35, and 45 in them; the only difference is the placement of the decimal and the 7 in the pH value. Otherwise, they have the same 35, and 45. This will help to remember these key values better.

3. Compensation of ABGS via the respiratory system: Always remember that the respiratory system blows off excess CO2 as a way to lower pH. To remember the pH and CO2 relationship: think of CO2 on one end of a sea-saw and pH on the other end. When pH is high, CO2 is low; therefore, the lungs will retain CO2. Also, when pH is low, CO2 is high; therefore, the lungs will blow off CO2.

4. Compensation of ABGS via the metabolic system: If pH is low, resulting in acidosis, the kidneys retain HCO3 (Sodium Bicarbonate). To remember pH and HCO3 relationship think of both the pH and HCO3 being in an elevator: when pH goes up, HCO3 goes up; likewise, when pH goes down HCO3 goes down, just like they are both riding an elevator.

5. Alkalosis or Acidosis has a low pH? Just use the alphabet to remember this: Acidosis is lower in a dictionary than Alkalosis is. In other words, Acidosis is lower in the dictionary alphabetically, than is Acidosis. Result: Acidosis is a low pH (below 7.35), while Alkalosis is a high pH (above 7.45).

Three hints for ABGs interpretation.

Normal blood pH is 7.35 to 7.45. The normal HCO3 is
21-28. Metabolic acidosis is a condition where the
blood pH is below 7.35 and the HCO3 is below 21.

To remember the things that can cause bicarbonate
(HCO3) to go down, below 21, think of the words,
CARB DOWN

C- Can be lowered with some antibiotics A- Aspirin or alcohol abuse R- Recurring diarrhea B- Burns D- Diabetes that is uncontrolled O- Overactive thyroid (i.e., hyperthyroidism) W- With liver or kidney disease N- Nutrition that is poor	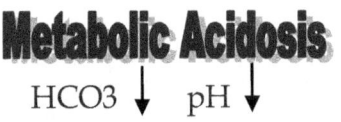 HCO3 ↓ pH ↓

Metabolic Alkalosis

During Metabolic alkalosis, the blood pH is high, above 7.45 and the sodium bicarbonate is high, above 28.

To remember the reasons that bicarbonate (HCO_3) goes up, think of the words CARB UP, as a shorter phrase for bicarbonate is up.

C- Corticosteroids A- Antacids R- Respiratory conditions such as COPD B- Blood transfusions U- Use of diuretics P- Persistent vomiting	**Metabolic Alkalosis** $HCO3 \uparrow \quad pH \uparrow$

Respiratory Alkalosis

During respiratory alkalosis the patient will have a CO_2 level below 22mm/L. To remember the conditions that can cause the CO_2 to go down and cause respiratory alkalosis think of the phrase carbon dioxide is down, then shorten it to the words, CARBON.

C- Cirrhosis A- Aspirin overdose R- Respiratory problems, i.e., pneumonia B- Bowel problems such as diarrhea O- Over ventilation, i.e., hyperventilation N- Not eating, i.e., starvation	Respiratory Alkalosis $CO_2 \downarrow$ $pH \uparrow$

Respiratory Acidosis

During respiratory acidosis the patient will have a CO_2 level below above 29mm/L. To remember the conditions that can cause the CO_2 to go up leading to respiratory acidosis think of the words respiratory acidosis, then shorten it to the word, ACIDOSIS.

A- Alcoholism C- COPD I- Increased or persistent vomiting D- Disorders such as Cushing's syndrome	Respiratory Acidosis $CO_2 \uparrow$ $pH \downarrow$

Causes of Hypokalemia

Hypokalemia is a conditionof low potassium in the body. Therefore, to remember the causes of hypokalemia, use a shorter version of the word potassium as in this: "POTAS"

> P- Potassium intake is low
> O- Oliguria
> T- Taking diuretics
> A- Aldosterone excess
> S- Secretions of the GI tract being lost

Signs and Symptoms of Hypokalemia

To remember the signs and symptoms of hypokalemia use word, "WEAKNESS" since it is one of the symptoms.

W- Weakness (lethargic)
E- Electrolytes may be abnormal
A- An absence of reflexes
K- K (potassium) will be below 3.5 mg/dl
N- Numbness
E- Extreme irritability of GI tract
S- Shortness of breath (SOB)
S- ST depression (as seen on ECG readings)

Signs and Symptoms of Hyperkalemia

To remember the signs and symptoms and treatment of hyperkalemia, use the word: "HYPER KALEMIA" broken into two words, one for S/S and one for treatment as seen below.

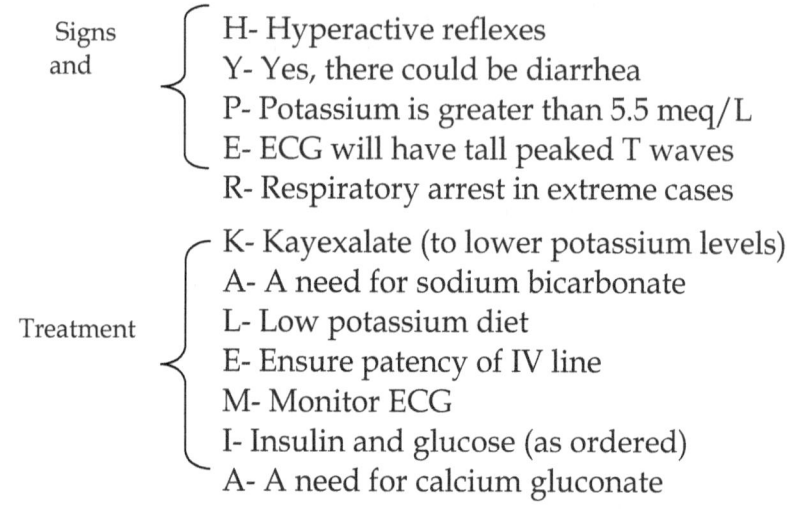

Signs and

H- Hyperactive reflexes
Y- Yes, there could be diarrhea
P- Potassium is greater than 5.5 meq/L
E- ECG will have tall peaked T waves
R- Respiratory arrest in extreme cases

Treatment

K- Kayexalate (to lower potassium levels)
A- A need for sodium bicarbonate
L- Low potassium diet
E- Ensure patency of IV line
M- Monitor ECG
I- Insulin and glucose (as ordered)
A- A need for calcium gluconate

Signs and Symptoms of Hypocalcemia

Since one of the primary signs and symptoms of hypocalcemia is tetany, to remember the signs and symptoms of hypocalcemia, use the word, "TETANY"

T- Tetany
E- ECG will reveal prolonged QT
T- Tingling
A- Arrhythmias
N- Numbness
Y- Your patient may have seizures in extreme cases

Treatment of Hypocalcemia

To remember the treatments of hypocalcemia think of the first syllable in the word calcium, namely, "CAL"

C- Calcium in diet
A- A need to correct underlying problem
L- Likely that patient will be on oral calcium

Signs and Symptoms of Hypercalcemia

Since bone pain is one of the signs and symptoms of hypercalcemia, to remember the signs and symptoms of this condition use the words, "BONE PAIN"

B- Bone pain
O- Oral membranes dry
N- Nausea and Constipation
E- Extremely tired

P- Possible heart block
A- Anorexia
I- Interval of QT shortened on ECG
N- Neuro reflexes slowed

Treatments of Hypercalcemia

To remember the treatments of Hypercalcemia think of three C's

    C- Correct underlying cause
    C- Calcium low in diet
    C- Corticosteroids

Causes of Hypophosphatemia

Hypophosphatemia is a condition of low phosphorus below 3.0 mg/dl. Since alcohol is one of the causes of Hypophosphatemia, think of the word, "ALCOHOL" to remember the causes of this condition.

    A- Alcohol abuse
    L- Loads of carbohydrates
    C- Chronic use of antacids
    O- Overly diuresis
    H- Hyper-alimentation
    O- Overly mechanical ventilation
    L- Loss of food absorption

Signs and Symptoms of Hypophosphatemia

Since one of the signs and symptoms and treatment of Hypophosphatemia is malaise, to remember the S/S of this condition use the word, "MALAISE".

M- Malaise and/or Muscle weakness
A- Anorexia
L- Low calcium diet
A- Assess LOC and neurological status
I- Irritability
S- Seizures
E- Encourage a diet high in phosphorus

Dialysis: Patient Management

Dialysis is a treatment to filter and clean blood. Therefore, to remember patient management for dialysis use the word, "FILTER"

F- Fistula, shunt should be assessed each shift for bruit
I- I/O hourly
L- Lund sounds every 4 hours (q4h)
T- Take vital signs every 15 min at the onset of treatment
E- Experiences of cramping during treatment--→ administer saline to decrease rate of dialysis
R- Reduce dialysis if patient develops Nausea, vomiting, or headache

Signs and Symptoms of

Hypomagnesemia

To remember the signs and symptoms and treatment of hypomagnesemia use the word, "MAGAZINE".

M- Magnesium will be less than 1.5 meq/L
A- Anorexia
G- Grapefruit, oranges and seafood are high in magnesium
A- Assess for signs of hypocalcemia
Z- Z as in ZZZ (to indicate need for rest)
I- IV magnesium (as ordered)
N- Nausea
E- Energy should be conserved (Rationale: patients often have muscle weakness)

Chapter 10-

Psychology Nursing

Bipolar Disorder: Manic Phase

A patient with Bipolar disorder will often have extreme mood changes going from mania to depression and back. The mood swings can be considered extreme. Therefore, to remember the signs and symptoms of bipolar disorder during the manic phase use the word: EXCITED

E- Euphoria

X- X as in eXtra shopping sprees

C- Can have inflated self-esteem

I- Impulsiveness

T- Thoughts that are racing

E- Excessive talk

D- Delusions

Bipolar Disorder: Depressive Phase

Conversely, to remember the signs and symptoms of bipolar disorder during the depressive phase use the word: DEPRESS as in the word depressed.

D- Depressed mood
E- Energy levels are low
P- Poor concentration
R- Results in lack of interest in usual activities
E- Extreme amounts of sleep or possibly insomnia
S- Sadness
S- Suicidal thoughts

Treatment of Bipolar Disorder

To remember the treatment of Bipolar Disorder you should use the word: LATE. As in don't wait too late to intervene.

L- Lithium
A- Antidepressants and/or Antipsychotic meds
T- Treatment during manic phase may require hospitalization
E- Electroconvulsive therapy (ECT) in extreme cases

Signs and Symptoms of Glaucoma

Glaucoma occurs from intraocular pressure increasing. Therefore, to remember the signs and symptoms of glaucoma remember the word: PRESSURE

> P- Pain in the eye
> R- Redness in eye
> E- Eye that looks hazy
> S- Seeing halos around lights
> S- Some loss of vision
> U- Uneasy stomach (ie. Nausea, Vomiting)
> R- Reduced vision: Tunnel vision
> E- Eye has pain

Signs and Symptoms of Bulimia

Patients with Bulimia will often not feel full. Therefore, to remember the signs and symptoms of bulimia use the words, NOT FULL.

N- Not regular menstrual periods

O- Overeating and feeling ashamed about it

T- Teeth marks on back of hands from inducing vomiting

F- Food is hidden is the house or other place

U- Usually talks about dieting, their weight, or body shape

L- Lack of energy

L- Lots of exercising to get rid of calories

Treatment of Bulimia

Patients who have bulimia will have to get control of their bulimia by getting medical attention. Therefore, to remember the treatments of bulimia use the word CONTROL.

C- Cognitive behavior therapy (may be needed)

O- Obsessive compulsive disorder may be a precipitating factor

N- Nutritional counseling

T- Three meals and two snacks a day and avoid unhealthy diets

R- Reduce concerns about patients body weight and shape

O- Other tests to test for signs of malnutrition

L- Liquids to prevent dehydration

Chapter 11- Cancer

Risk factors of Prostate Cancer

To remember the risk factors for prostate cancer, remember one of the risk factors, which is RACE

> R- Race (African Americans have higher incidence)
> A- Age
> C- Can be hereditary
> E- Exercise: a lack of exercise

Signs and Symptoms of Prostate Cancer

To remember the signs and symptoms of prostate cancer use the word: FREQUENT

F- Frequency

R- Reduced weight and appetite (in advanced
  stages)

E- Examination (Digital Rectal Exam)

Q- Question patient as to whether they have
  pain in pelvis

U- Urinary stream is weak

E- Elevated PSA (prostate specific antigen) levels

N- Nausea and vomiting (in advanced stages)

T- Tumor within prostate

Side Effects of Chemotherapy

To remember the most common temporary side effects
of chemotherapy, use the word: HAIR LOSS

> H- Hair loss
> A- Appetite loss
> I- Infertility
> R- Reduced immunity

> L- Low white blood cell count
> O- Other side effects include low platelet count
> S- Sores in mouth
> S- Side effects related to chemotherapy will go
>   away once treatment is stopped

Assessment Findings of Neutropenia

Neutropenia is a decreased production of neutrophils, one of the white blood cells. To remember the WBC's of the body and some of the assessment findings of Neutropenia think of the word, "BENEFIT" since white blood cells benefit the body by fighting off infections.

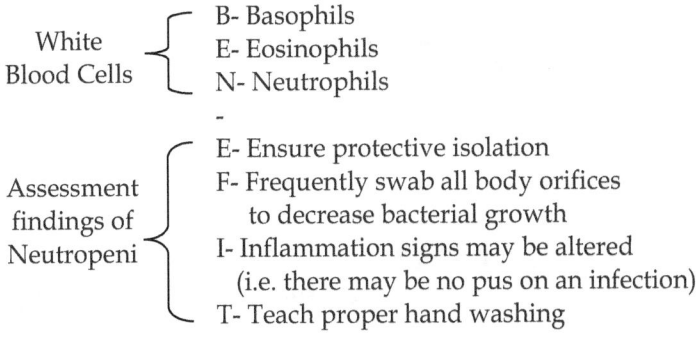

White
Blood Cells
B- Basophils
E- Eosinophils
N- Neutrophils

-

Assessment
findings of
Neutropeni
E- Ensure protective isolation
F- Frequently swab all body orifices
    to decrease bacterial growth
I- Inflammation signs may be altered
    (i.e. there may be no pus on an infection)
T- Teach proper hand washing

Chapter 12-

Miscellaneous

Signs and Symptoms of Benign Prostatic Hypertrophy

Benign Prostatic Hypertrophy (BPH) is a very serious condition of the prostate; many men can develop it as they get older. Since BPH is a BENIGN condition, (and is the B in the abbreviation BPH), use it to remember the signs and symptoms of BPH.

> B- Beginning urine stream is slow
> E- Extra trips to bathroom: (i.e. frequent urination)
> N- Nocturia
> I- Impossible to urinate if bladder stones block ureters
> G- Greater age (50 years old or older) more likely to occur
> N- Need to urinate frequently

Treatments of Benign Prostatic Hypertrophy

Since one of the treatments of BPH is Trans Urethral Resection of Prostate (TURP) and the BPH has the word HyperTROPHY in it, use the word TROPHY to remember the treatments of BPH.

T- TransUrethral
R- Resection
O- Of

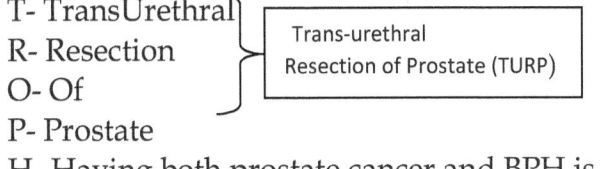

Trans-urethral
Resection of Prostate (TURP)

P- Prostate
H- Having both prostate cancer and BPH is possible
Y- Yearly screening for prostate cancer should continue after pt. treated for BPH

Signs and Symptoms of Shingles

Shingles is a condition that has rash associated with it. Therefore, to remember the signs and symptoms of Shingles use the word: RASH

R- Rash
A- A feeling of tingling and itching
S- Stabbing pain on the skin
H- Having fluid filled blisters that crust over after a few days

Signs and Symptoms of Osteoarthritis

Osteoarthritis can cause the bones to rub together and lead to friction. Since this rubbing of bones can happen, use the word FRICTION to remember the signs and symptoms and treatment.

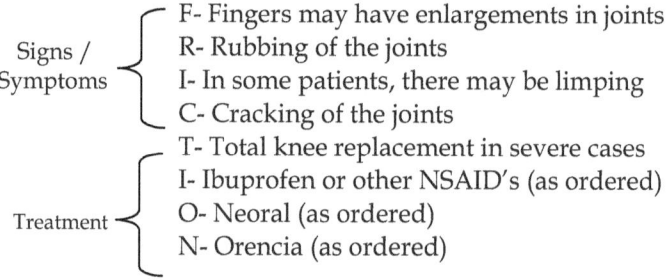

Signs / Symptoms
- F- Fingers may have enlargements in joints
- R- Rubbing of the joints
- I- In some patients, there may be limping
- C- Cracking of the joints

Treatment
- T- Total knee replacement in severe cases
- I- Ibuprofen or other NSAID's (as ordered)
- O- Neoral (as ordered)
- N- Orencia (as ordered)

Signs and Symptoms of Alzheimer' s Disease

To remember the signs and symptoms of Alzheimer's think of LOST as it is one of the symptoms.

L- Lost in places the patient usually knows well
O- Often eats poorly
S- Same questions asked repeatedly
T- Taking care of oneself is difficult

ADHD Signs and Symptoms

Attention deficit hyperactivity disorder (ADHD) is a condition in which patients have excessive hyperactivity. To remember the signs and symptoms and some treatment of ADHD use the word: HYPERACTIVE

H- Hyperactivity

Y- Yes, behavior does change with age: children are often more restless

P- Performing and completing tasks is usually difficult

E- Exact cause is not clear, but is does tend to run in families

R- Ritalin (as ordered)

A- Adderall

C- Concerta (as ordered)

T- There is no cure but treatment can control symptoms

I- Impulsiveness

V- Very inattentive

E- Enjoying task like reading are difficult for ADHD patients

Symptoms of Chronic Fatigue Syndrome

One of the main symptoms of chronic fatigue syndrome (CFS) is long-term fatigue. Therefore to remember the signs and symptoms of CFS use the word, FATIGUE.

> F- Forgetfulness
> A- A headache that is different from other headaches in the past
> T- Tender lymph nodes
> I- Increase in heart rate and decrease in BP (i.e. orthostatic hypotension)
> G- Gradually develops over weeks or months (in some cases)
> U- Unrested- usually wake up tired
> E- Extended period of tiredness that lasts longer than 6 months

Smoke Inhalation

To remember one of the key signs of smoke inhalation use the word, "SMOKE".

S- Sounds from lungs will reveal crackles

M- May have carbonaceous sputum

O- 0 2 levels will be low

K- Knocked out possible (as in fainting, seizures, or coma)

E- Elevated CO2 levels

Disseminated Intravascular Coagulation

Disseminated Intravascular Coagulation (DIC) is a condition that has low platelet count. Since it involves low platelet count, think of the word, "PLATELETS" when you think of the signs and symptoms of DIC.

P- PT time will be greater than 15 seconds

L- Low platelet count

A- Anxious

T- Tachycardia

E- Elevated Respiratory Rate

L- Low urine output (Oliguria)

E- Ecchymoses

T- Tender abdomen

S- Some bleeding from multiple orifices and mucus membranes

Treatment of DIC

To remember the treatment of DIC use the phrase:
"GIVE BLOOD"

>G- Gasses should be monitored (i.e. ABG's)
>I- Implement cold compresses
>V- Vital signs every 15 min
>E- Established clots should not be disturbed

>B- Blood administered (as ordered)
>L- LOC monitored
>O- O2 (as ordered)
>O- Oximetry (i.e. pulse oximetry)
>D- Dopamine (as ordered) to enhance
>   contractility

Signs and Symptoms of Septic Shock

A gram negative bacterial infections can be one of the most common causes of septic shock. To remember the S/S of septic shock use the word, "BACTERIAL"

B- Blood pressure will be low
A- Anxiety
C- Cool clammy skin
T- Temperature will be high
E- Evidence of multiple organ failure
R- Rapid respirations
I- Increased heart rate
A- A weak thready pulse
L- Low urine output (oliguria)

Treatment of Septic Shock

To remember the treatment of septic shock use the word, "DOPAMINE" since it is one of the treatments.

D- Dopamine (as ordered)
O- Oxygen (as ordered)
P- Phenylephrine
A- Antibiotics
M- Mechanical ventilation
I- Inotropes (i.e. dobutamine)
N- Norepinephrine
E- Evaluate patients vital signs

Symptoms and Complications of Blood Transfusions

To remember the signs and symptoms of complications of a blood transfusion, use the acronym from one of the symptoms: "FEBRILE"

> F- Febrile
> E- Excessive fluid
> B- Brain hurts (if there is fluid overload)
> R- Really short of breath (SOB)
> I- Ineffective breathing
> L- Lumbar region pain
> E- Excessive central venous pressure (CVP)

Treatment and Precautions After Surgery

Treatment and precautions of patient after surgery-→ Some patients may require gastric surgery since many will have an NG tube after surgery. To remember the patient management for gastric surgery associate it with the words, "NG

TUBE" .

Treatmen ⎰ N- NG Tube
         ⎱ G- Give O2 (as ordered)

Things to
report to
physician
          ⎰ T- Temperature elevations or signs
          ⎮   of infection
          ⎮ U- Uncontrolled pain
          ⎮ B- BP or other V/S that are decreasing
          ⎱ E- Excreting less than 30 ml/hr

Assessment and Treatment of Head Injuries

To remember the assessment / treatment of head injuries think of one of the interventions for this condition, "CHECK LOC".

C- Check level of consciousness (LOC) frequently

H- Head of bead (HOB) elevated

E- Ear and nose checked and monitored for drainage

C- Check vital signs frequently

K- Keep a quiet environment

-

L- Liquids should be restricted (to help lower ICP)

O- Output and input monitored

C- CT scan (as ordered)

Signs and Symptoms & Treatment of Head Injuries

To remember how to the signs and symptoms and treatment of head injuries remember this word association: BRAIN

B- Bradycardia may be present

R- Raise HOB 30 degrees

A- Assess LOC

I- Increased Intracranial pressure (ICP)

N- Need to reduce cerebral edema with osmotic diuretics

Treatment of Chest Trauma

To remember the treatment of Chest Trauma use the word association: COLLAPSE as in a collapsed lung.

C- Chest tube insertion
O- Oxygen
L- Lungs may need mechanical ventilation
L- Lungs should be monitored for any
    adventitious sounds
A- A recording of chest drainage hourly
P- PEEP may be used
S- Stabilize chest wall
E- Epidural analgesics

Amblyopia

Amblyopia, is a condition of lazy eye. To remember the treatment of this condition, use a word from one of the treatments, "PATCH"

P- Patch the healthy eye
A- Assess for central vision loss in suppressed
    eye
T- Treat child before age 6
C- Can lead to vision loss from disuse
H- Have breaks from wearing patch (this keeps
    strong eye from becoming weakened

Chapter 13- List of Additional NCLEX-RN Study Tips

Additional NCLEX-RN Study Tips	
Topic	Tip
1) Smoking and Alcoholism: "Smoking has a C in cigarettes; bottle has a b in it"	**Alcoholism and smoking and their need for certain Vitamins** For a patient with alcoholism, they will have an increase need for vitamin B; think of B and Bottle. In a patient that smokes, they will have an increase need for vitamin C. Think of C in the word cigarettes, and associate it with smoking.

2) Treatment for congestive heart failure (CHF): "Unload"	**Treatment for congestive heart failure** Think of the acronym UNLOAD: U for upright position; N nitrates; L for low sodium diet; O for oxygen; A for reducing anxiety (Morphine sulfate); D for Digitalis.
3) When assessing a patient with chest pain, think of: "LID"	**Assessing a patient with chest pain** When assessing patients with chest pain use the following phrase: "Did you check the LID?" L- Location- Suspect a MI is the patient complains of sub-sternal pain radiating to arm, jaw, or back. I- Intensity - D- Duration - Sudden onset of pain that is ongoing suggests MI

4) Precipitating factors for Myocardial Infarction: "SEAT"	**Precipitating factors for Myocardial Infarction** Precipitating factors for Myocardial Infarction (MI), think of the following: "It is sweet for the patient to take a SEAT." S -Stress E - Eating too much A - Anxiety T- Temperature changes
5) Medications used to treat Myocardial Infarction: "BUILT"	**Medications used to treat Myocardial Infarction** Medications used to treat Myocardial Infarction (MI) and angina can be remembered by using this phrase: "There will be no guilt when you think BUILT." B- Blocadren U- Urokinase I- Inderal L- Lopressor T- Tenormin

6) Teaching patients how to prevent coronary artery disease: "HOCUS"	**Teaching instructions for Coronary Artery Disease** Teaching patients how to prevent coronary artery disease (CAD) isn't as easy as hocus pocus, but you can remember it by using the acronym HOCUS: H- Hypertension/and hyperlipedmia O- Obesity C- Cocaine use U- Uncontrolled diabetes S- Sedentary lifestyle/ and smoking.
7) Thrombolytic Enzymes used in patients with acute Myocardial Infarction: "USA"	**Medications used in patients Myocardial Infarction** Medications used in patients with acute Myocardial Infarction (MI) are Thrombolytic Enzymes. To remember these think in this manner: "USA is the only way." U- Urokinase S- Streptokinase A- Alteplase

8) PT for coumadin *"PT for play therapy and children"*	**PT and PTT** In Prothombin Time (PT) associate the *PT with play therapy; in play therapy think of children* and therefore Coumadin and children (both have the letter c). When Coumadin is used on a client, the PT values will increase. In Partial Thoromboplastin Time (PTT) think of the other anticoagulant: heparin. When heparin is used it will increase the PTT values. Values: PTT normal is 68-82 PT normal is 11-15 (associate the *c in coumadin for children and think of play therapy and you get PT.* *Think of 11-15 as the range of children while in play therapy.*

9) Aruptio Placenta and Placenta Previa *"Think of going to a movie."*	**Placenta Previa/ Abuptio Placenta** Think of placenta previa as a movie preview (think: previa as a preview).| In a movie preview, you may see *blood* on the screen; you will be seated on a *soft* seat, and you will have *no pain*. The clinical manifestations for placenta previa are: *blood, soft abdomen, and no pain*. Therefore, in aruptio placenta, the symptoms are just the opposite: no blood, rigid abdomen, and pain.
	Anti-Anxiety Medications Normally, we think of "smelling the roses" as a way to relax. In thinking of anti-anxieties, think of "smelling the LEAVES" as a way to relax: L- Librium; E- Equanil; *A*- Ativan; V- Valium; E- Equanil S- Serax.

Topic	Tip
11) When dealing with patients with dementia: "RISE"	**Dementia** When dealing with patients with dementia (Parkinson's Alzheimer's or any form of dementia) always think "we want them to RISE in the morning: *R*- eality: Bring them back to reality. *I*-ndependence - Maintain independence with them *S*-elf esteem - Improve their self-esteem *E*-nvironment- Provide precautions for patitient on photosensitive medications; provide safety-especially for those on tranquilizers.
12)	**Hegar's Sign**

Hegar's Sign	Think "hey you": hey-for hegars and you-for uterus Hegar's sign is a softening of the uterus during pregnancy
13) Diagnostic tests of colorectal cancer can be remembered by using: "DEAF"	**Diagnostic tests for colorectal cancer** Diagnostic tests of colorectal cancer can be remembered by using this acronym: DEAF. D- Digital Rectal Exam: can detect 15% of colorectal cancers. E- Excretory urography: to verify function and displacement of kidneys, ureters, or bladder by a tumor pressing against them. A- Antigen Carcinoembryonic: permits patient monitoring before and after treatment. F- Fecal occult blood test: can detect blood in stools

14) Causes of Cor pulmonale: "COLT"	**Causes of Cor pulmonale:** Cor Pulmonale doesn't need to be a jolt to think of Colt: use COLT to remember the causes of Cor pulmonale. C- COPD / and Cystic Fibrosis O- Obesity L- Living at high altitude T- Tuberculosis These all increase the heart's workload and lead to right side hypertrophy.
15) Treatment of Cor pulmonale: "SODA"	**Treatment of Cor pulmonale (right-sided heart failure)** The signs and symptoms of Cor pulmonale can be remembered by using the acronym SODA: S- Sputum Culture O- O2 administration D- Digoxin A- Antibiotics: to treat any underlying respiratory infection.

16) Signs and symptoms of Polycythemia Vera: "DEPART"	**Signs and symptoms of Polycythemia Vera:** Polycythemia Vera is an excess production of RBC's. This excess of RBC in circulation leads to the following signs and symptoms that can be remembered by using the acronym DEPART in this phrase: "If the excess red blood cells (RBC's) would DEPART, then the patient would not have polycythemia vera." D- Dizziness E- Epigastric pain P- Pleuritic chest pain A- Abdominal fullness R- Rushing in the ears T- Tinnitus
17) Treatment of Polycythemia Vera: "CAP"	**Treatment of Polycythemia Vera:** To remember treatments for Polycythemia Vera don't Nap, just use the acronym CAP. C- Chemotherapy: melphalan, busulfan, chlorambucil. A- Allopurinol: to treat the uric acid

	levels. P- Phlebotomy: used to reduce the RBC buildup.
18) Preventing Thrombophlebitis: "WALK"	**Preventing Thrombophlebitis** Deep vein thrombosis is the thrombosis of deep veins which can occur postoperatively due to immobility. A complication of DVT is pulmonary embolism. To remember treatments to prevent DVT postoperatively use the acronym: WALK W- Warfarin sodium (Coumadin) A- Ambulation / and Anti-embolism stockings (TED hose) L- Lipohepin (Heparin sodium) K- Keep extremity elevated
19) Signs and symptoms of Hypoglycemia: "DIETETIC"	**Signs and symptoms of Hypoglycemia:** During insulin administration the diabetic patient it prone to insulin shock (hypoglycemia). To remember the signs/symptoms of hypoglycemia think of the word

DIETETIC
in this phrase: "The diabetic must watch for DIETETIC."

D- Diaphoresis

I- Irritability

E- Excess food intake

T- Tachycardia

E- Extreme weakness

T- Tremors

I- Irregular speech (i.e.: slurred speech)

C- Clammy skin

20)

Peritonitis

"R in Peritonitis is for rigid and rebound"

Peritonitis

"*Associate the r in Peri with rigid and rebound*"

A patient with Peritonitis will have a rigid abdomen, rebound tenderness, and decreased bowel sounds.

Topic	Tip
21) Sickle cell crisis *"Think sick cells"*	**Sickle cell crisis** Sickle cell crisis occurs from dehydration, lack of oxygen, and acidosis. (*Think of the cells being sick and needing: oxygen, water, and normal ph levels*).
22) Allergic Reaction to a Blood Transfusion: "CRAFT"	**Allergic Reaction to a Blood Transfusion** To remember allergic reactions to a blood transfusion think of the following phrase: "administering blood is a CRAFT." C-Chills / Chest pain R- Restlessness A- Apprehension F- Fever / Flushing of skin T- Tachycardia
23) When assessing for Mitral valve	**Mitral valve stenosis** When assessing for Mitral valve stenosis think of the following phrase:

stenosis: "SMALLER"	"The opening is SMALLER". S- Secondary CHF M- Mitral valve stiffens and does not open normally A- Adventitious (see next one) L- Lung sounds L- Loud S1 E- Edema (peripheral edema secondary to CHF) R- Rheumatic Fever: Rheumatic fever can lead to mitral valve stenosis
24) Atropine contraindicated in patients with glaucoma. "Glaucoma and *Atropine* are *not keen* together"	**Atropine contraindicated in patients with glaucoma.** Atropine is contraindicated in patients with glaucoma; anticholinergic drugs, like atropine, produce pupil dilation causing impaired outflow of aqueous humor from the eye. A phrase to remember that atropine is contraindicated in patients with glaucoma use the one below: "Glaucoma and *Atropine* are *not keen* together"

25) Clinical manifestations of pyelonephritis: "CLUE"	**Clinical manifestations of pyelonephritis** To remember the signs and symptoms of pyelonephritis use the phrase: "get a clue with pyelonephritis". C- Chills and fever L- Lower flank pain U- Urinary frequency E- Elevated WBC's
26) Clinical manifestations of cystitis: "UPP"	**Clinical manifestations of cystitis** Since patients with cystitis have urinary frequency, the best way to remember the signs and symptoms of cystitis is to think of the letters: U.P.P U- Urinary frequency P- Pain in groin and lower abdomen P- Pain during urination
27) Clinical manifestations of Peritonitis: "GLASS"	**Clinical manifestations of Peritonitis** To remember the signs and symptoms of peritonitis use the following phrase: when a patient has Peritonitis it may feel like they have "GLASS in their

	stomach"
	G- Generally constipated
	L- Low grade fever
	A- Absent bowel sounds
	S- Shallow respirations
	S- Sever abdominal pain
28) Complications of Cirrhosis: "AGREE"	**Complications of Cirrhosis** Cirrhosis of the liver can be caused by malnutrition, viral hepatitis, and alcohol abuse/use. To remember the complications of Hepatic Cirrhosis use the following phrase: Heavy alcohol consumption does not "AGREE" with patients. A- Ascites G- GI Bleeding R- Retention of water E- Encephalopathy (from the high levels of ammonia buildup) E- Esophageal Varices

29)

Interventions for Ulcerative Colitis:

"VIBRANT"

Interventions for Ulcerative Colitis

Use this phrase to remember the interventions for patients with ulcerative colitis are not very VIBRANT

V- Vitamin and mineral supplement

I- Intake and output (monitor I & O)

B- Bed rest

R- Relieve pain

A- Antibiotics/ and antiemetics

N- Nutritional support: TPN

T- Turn every 2 hours

30)

Potassium Chloride

POTASSIUM CHLORIDE

Never give Potassium Chloride (KCl) IV push or IM. This is a lethal injection. It must be diluted and administered by IV drip.

Topic	Tip
31) Mixing Regular and NPH Insulin: "RN"	**Think of Registered nurse (RN) when mixing Insulin:** R for Regular and N for NPH insulin. When giving both types, draw up the regular first then the NPH. This prevents contamination. Also, remember that the *mixture should be given within 5 minutes*. Waiting longer than 5 minutes will result in a breakdown of the regular insulin by the NPH leading to a weak acting formula.

| 32)

Tips for ABG's:

"Buy A Car" | **Tips for ABG's**

Normal levels of ABG's:

(pH: 7.35-7.45) (Normal CO2 is 35-45) (Normal HCO3 is 22-26)

Hint 1: Normal pH: 7.35-7.45. Note: Notice that both CO2 and pH have some of the same numbers: 3, 5 and 4, 5 in them. (See Co2 below)

Hint 2: Normal CO2 is 35-45. Useful tip: It has some of the same numbers that normal pH has: 7.35-7.45

Hint 3: Normal HCO3 is 22-26. Use this tip:

Suppose an auto driver buys their first car between 22 -26 y/o. Therefore, think of sodium bicarbonate as sodium "Buy-A-carbonate", or bicarbonate as in sodium bicarbonate. |
| 33)

Positive Guthrie tests:

"LEGS" | **Positive Guthrie tests**

To remember when Guthrie tests are positive use this acronym: LEGS.

Guthrie tests are used to screen for deficiency of phenylalanine hydroxylase, and enzyme that converts phenylalanine to tyrosine in infants. |

Too much phenylalanine can lead to mental retardation. The Guthrie test will identify this deficiency. Also, remember that Guthrie test will be elevated when:

Guthrie tests are positive when: LEGS

L- Low birth weight

E- Encephalopathy

G- Galactosemia

S- Septicemia

Also, PKU can lead to a positive Guthrie test.

---

34)

Serum Amylase Levels increased:

"DRAB"

Serum Amylase Levels Increased

Serum Amylase Levels- are elevated in patients with pancreatitis. Below are acronyms to remember when it is increased or decreased:

Amylase Elevated: (DRAB)

D- Diabetic acidosis

R- Renal failure

A- Acute pancreatitis

B- BHP (Benign Prostatic Hypertrophy)

"CASH is down, DRAB is up."

35) Amylase Levels Decreased: "CASH"	**Amylase Levels Decreased** C- Chronic A- Alcoholism S- Severe Burns H- Hepatitis "CASH is down, DRAB is up."
36) Bronchodilators: "A DIET"	**Bronchodilators** Bronchodilators used in respiratory conditions to open breathing passages by dilating bronchioles to relieve bronchospasms. Bronchodilators usually cause decreased appetite; so, use "A Diet" as an acronym to remember the Bronchodilators. (A Diet) A- Albuterol D- Dyphylline I- Isoproterenol E- Epinephrine T- Theophylline

37) Meds that cause false negative Thyroxine Serum level: "PILOT"	**Meds that cause false negative level Thyroxine Serum** Thyroxine Serum (T-4) is used to determine thyroid function. A. Drugs that cause false negatives can be thought of with the acronym PILOT: P- Phenytoin (Dilantin) I- Inderal L- Lithium O- Orinase T- Thorazine
38) Meds that cause a false positive Thyroxine Serum level: "CEO"	**Meds that cause false positive level Thyroxine Serum** Thyroxine Serum (T-4) is used to determine thyroid function. Meds that cause false positive can be thought of with the acronym CEO (as in CEO of a company). C- Clofibrate E- Estrogen O- Oral Contraceptives

39) White Blood Cells (WBC's): "BEN"	**White Blood Cells (WBC's)** Using BEN to remember White Blood Cells: Use Acronym "BEN" when remembering the types of White Blood Cells (Leukocytes): The three types of leukocytes are best remembered by using the acronym BEN: B- Basophils E- Eosinophils N- Neutrophils
40) Cardinal signs of Diabetes mellitus "Use a Dip -er to get water" "G is for gas in the stomach"	**Cardinal signs of Diabetes:** 1. Poly**dip**sia-(Excessive thirst) associate "**dip**" with dipping for water, as in using a dipper to get water. 2. Polypha**g**ia (excessive hunger) associate "**g**" with gas and the stomach. This will help to associate polyphagia with excessive hunger 3. Polyuria (excessive urination) These are key assessment findings of diabetes.

Topic	Tip
41) (BUN) 8-25mg/dl "Hotdog BUN"	**Blood Urea Nitrogen (BUN) Level** Blood Urea Nitrogen (BUN) is a byproduct of metabolism. An elevated BUN is a sign of dehydration, renal failure, or GI bleeding. A key tip to remember the normal level is: Think of the junk food that most people in the **8-25 y/o age group eat**: hamburgers, hot dogs. Then associate it with hotdog buns and hamburger buns. Thus, **8-25**mg/dl is the normal BUN range.
42) Assessment of Alcoholism "5 D's"	**Assessment of Alcoholism** When assessing for alcoholism: (Think of 5 D's) D- Denial

	D- Dependent D- Demanding D- Dissatisfied D- Domineering
43) S/S of of Hodgkin's disease: "ELF"	**Signs and Symptoms of Hodgkin's disease** For Signs/Symptoms of Hodgkin's disease use the acronym ELF: E- Enlarged L- Lymph Nodes F- Fever (Slight to High Fever)
44) ESR is low when: "SPACE"	**Erythrocyte Sedimentation Rate (ESR Rate) low** Erythrocyte Sedimentation Rate (ESR Rate) is the rate RBC's settle out of unclotted blood. Use the word Spaceship and the phrase: "Space is low but the Ship is high in ESR." Levels of ESR are decreased during the following: (SPACE) S- Sickle Cell Anemia P- Polycythemia

	A- Angina Pectoris C- CHF E- Ethambutol (Patients taking Ethambutol)
45) ESR is high when: "SHIP"	**Erythrocyte Sedimentation Rate (ESR Rate) high** Levels of ESR are increased during the following: (SHIP) S- Surgery H- Hodgkin's Disease I- Infections P- Pregnancy (also in PID) To summarize ESR: "The Space is low but the Ship is high in ESR"
46) Management for Hodgkin's disease: "MOPP"	**Management for Hodgkin's disease** Management for Hodgkin's disease you can use the acronym MOPP: Chemotherapy used to treat Hodgkin's disease can be remembered using MOPP: M- Mustargen

	O- Oncovin P- Procarbazine P- Prednisone
47) Decreased Serum ALbumin: "SCAB"	**Decreased Serum Albumin** Serum Albumin is synthesized by the liver. A decrease in albumin results in edema. Normal levels are 3.5- 5.0g/dL. Decreased Levels of Albumin occur when: SCAB S- Sulfonamides (patients taking sulfonamides) C- Cirrhosis A- Aspirin B- Burns (Severe Burns)
48) Increased Serum Albumin: "DVD"	**Increased Serum Albumin** Levels of Albumin are increased during: DVD D- Dehydration V- Vomiting D- Diarrhea To summarize Albumin: "DVD is the

	Key to high albumin, and a SCAB will grab low albumin."
49) Glucose in CSF: "Is 2/3 that of blood glucose"	**Glucose in Cerebrospinal fluid** In blood glucose the normal range is 70-110 mg/DL. In Cerebrospinal fluid (CSF) glucose, the range is two-thirds that of blood glucose: 50-80mg/DL. In other words: two-thirds of 70 is 50 and two-thirds of 110 is 80.
50) Decreased LOC: "Dolls Eyes"	**Decreased LOC** Think of the eyes of a doll: when you move in front of the doll the eyes never move. In a patient with the low level of consciousness, you will see doll's eyes. The more they get "doll's eyes" the lower their level of consciousness is getting.

Topic	Tip
51) Fetal Monitoring: "Extension cords come in Variable lengths." "Being Late for appointments is insufficient"	**Fetal Monitoring** Variable decelerations are caused by cord compression. Hint: *Think of a cord coming in variable lengths, like an extension cord coming in variable lengths.* Associate the *variable lengths of cords* and you have **variable decelerations**. Variable decelerations means cord compression. Think of *being late for an appointment as insufficient:* Late deceleration is indicative of placental insufficiency.

52)

Decreased
Platelets:

"SLICK"

Decreased Platelets

Platelets: (150,000 uL- 400,000) uL.
Pltelets are the basic elements in blood
that promote coagulation.

Platelet levels are decreased during:
SLICK
"The trick with low platelets is to think
SLICK"

S- SLE

L- Liver Disease

I- Idiopathic thrombocytopenic purpura
(ITP)

C- Cancer

K- Kidney Disease

53) Increased Platelets : "SPAM"	**Increased Platelets** When Plaetlets are increased think: SPAM S- Splenectomy P- Polycythemia Vera A- Acute Blood Loss M- Myeloproliferative disorders To summarize Platelets: "SPAM I AM with High Platelets and the trick with low platelets is to think SLICK"

54)

How the fetus goes through the birth canal:

"Every darn fool in Egypt eats raw eggs"

How the fetus goes through the birth canal

Use the first letter of every word in this mnemonic to remember how the fetus goes through the birth canal use this phrase:

"Every darn fool in Egypt eats raw eggs."

E- Engagement.

D- Descent

F- Flexion

I- Internal

E- Extension

ER- External

E- Expulsion

55) Signs and Symptoms of Rocky Mountain spotted fever: "NAPPER"	**Signs and Symptoms of Rocky Mountain spotted fever:** To remember the signs and symptoms of Rocky Mountain spotted fever use the acronym NAPPER: N- Nagging Cough A- Abdominal Pain P- Persistent cough P- Pain in joint muscle, and back E- Excruciating Headache R- Rash To remember NAPPER use this phrase: "A NAPPER who naps in wooded areas may come in contact with ticks."

56) Diagnostic Tests of Rocky Mountain spotted fever: "PALLID"	**Diagnostic Tests of Rocky Mountain spotted fever** Use the acronym PALLID. P- Platelet count low A- Abnormal hepatic function L- Low Blood Count L- Latex Agglutination (A titer of 128 after 1 week onset.) I- Indirect Immunofluoresence (A titer of 64 or greater.) D- Decreased serum albumin
57) Treatment of Rocky Mountain spotted fever: "PART"	**Treatment of Rocky Mountain spotted fever** To remember the treatments of Rocky Mountain spotted fever use the acronym PART in the following manner: "Patients should not let a tick get on any PART of their body." P- Platelet count treatment A- Anti-seizure meds

	R- Removal of Tick very carefully T- Tetracycline
58) Nursing Interventions of Rocky Mountain spotted fever: "FAITH"	**Nursing Interventions of Rocky Mountain spotted fever** Use the acronym FAITH. F - Frequent turning of patient A - Administer analgesics I - I.V. Fluids T - Tepid sponge baths H - High-protein, high-calorie meals
59) 7 Warning signs of cancer: "CAUTION"	**7 Warning signs of cancer** Think of the word Caution: C -Change in bowel or bladder. A -A lesion that does not heal. U -Unusual bleeding or discharge. T -Thickening or difficult in swallowing. I -Indigestion or difficulty swallowing.

O -Obvious changes in wart or mole.

N - Nagging cough or persistent hoarseness.

60)

Signs of labor and delivery:

"WORLDS"

Signs of labor and delivery

Think of a fetus going out into the worlds:

W- Weight loss.

O- Opposite in sensations (like cramping in legs).

R- Rupture of the membrane.

L- Lightening.

D- Dilation and effacement.

S- Sudden burst of energy 24-48hrs. prior to labor.

Topic	Tip
61) Signs/symptoms of Cystic Fibrosis: "LIPASE"	**Signs/symptoms of Cystic Fibrosis** To remember the s/s of cystic fibrosis use this acronym:Lipase L- Lipase, amylase, and trypsin are decreased. I- Iontophoresis sweat test. P- Pancreatic Enzymes low. A- Airway obstructed from increased mucus production. S- Steatorrhea. E- Examine for distended abdomen.

62) Nursing Interventions of Cystic Fibrosis: "AMYLASE"	**Nursing Interventions of Cystic Fibrosis** For nursing interventions of Cystic Fibrosis use this acronym: Amylase A- Administer IV antibiotics M- Multivitamins, especially fat-soluble vitamins. Y- Young: Life-span into mid forties. L- Lavage of bronchi in some cases. A- Aerosol and expectorants to decrease viscosity of secretions. S- Salt intake: ensure adequate salt and fluid intake. E- Enzymes (pancreatic) given with meals.
63) Signs and Symptoms of Tuberculosis: "SHAFT"	**Signs and Symptoms of Tuberculosis** Use the following phrase to remember the signs and symptoms of Tuberculosis: "To remember signs and symptoms of Tuberculosis don't think of a draft, think of a SHAFT." S- Sweats at night.

	H- Hemoptysis.
	A- Anorexia.
	F- Fever (low grade).
	T- Tired (Fatigued).
64) Diagnostic Tests of Tuberculosis: "CHAP"	**Diagnostic Tests of Tuberculosis** Use this phrase to remember diagnostic tests for tuberculosis: "With Diagnostic tests for Tuberculosis you won't need a map. You just need to think of the word CHAP." C- Chest X-Ray. H- Hematology (increased WBC). A- Acid Bacilli is Positive. P- Positive culture for mycobacterium tuberculosis

65) Treatment of Tuberculosis: "CAD"	**Treatment of Tuberculosis** Use this phrase to remember treatment of Tuberculosis: "Treatment of TB is not so bad when you use the acronym CAD." C- Chest physiotherapy postural drainage (CPPD). A- Airborne Precautions. D- Diet high in carbohydrates and proteins.
66) Meds for Tuberculosis : "SHRIMP"	**Meds for Tuberculosis** Medications used to treat Tuberculosis are best remembered by using this phrase: "Tuberculosis need not make one Limp when you use the acronym SHRIMP. S- Streptomycin. H- Hepatic function monitoring. R- Rifampin. I- Isoniazide. M- Myambutol. P- Pyrazinamide.

67) Hypoglycemia: "Don't get upset unless they get wet."	**Hypoglycemia** When an insulin dependent diabetic goes into hypoglycemic shock, they will become diaphoretic. Check for wet sheets or wet clothing on this patient. Use this phrase to remember that low blood sugar: "Don't get upset unless they get wet." Low BS level needs immediate attention. It is easier to get a high BS down, than it is to get a low BS up.
68) Cystic Fibrosis "F is in failure to thrive and F is in cystic fibrosis."	**Cystic Fibrosis can cause failure to thrive** Use the F in failure to thrive and associate it with Fibrosis.

69)

Meds that suppress labor:

"BEVY"

Meds that suppress labor

To remember medicatios that suppress labor use this acronym: BEVY.

B- Brethine (Terbutaline)

E- Electrolytes monitored

V- Vasodilan (Isoxsuprine)

Y- Yutopar (Ritodrine)

Use this phrase to remember Bevy: "The mother will remain top-heavy when you use BEVY."

70)

Side effects of Pitocin

"PIT"

Side effects of Pitocin

Pitocin is used to induce labor. To remember the side effects of Pitocin think of the first syllable in Pitocin:PIT.

P -Pressure increased (Hypertension)

I - I/O monitoring

T - Titanic contractions

Topic	Tip
71) Dysphasia and Dysphagia "S for speaking and G for gas"	**Difference in Dysphasia and Dysphagia** To remember the difference in Dysphasia and Dysphagia, use this phrase: "Think of S for speaking and G for Gas in stomach." Therefore, dysphasia is difficulty in speaking. And, Dysphagia is difficulty in swallowing.
72) Procedures done after a lumbar puncture: "FRAM"	**Procedures after a lumbar puncture** To remember the nursing interventions after a lumbar puncture use this acronym: FRAM. F- Force fluids R- Record procedure, and appearance of spinal fluid A- Administer analgesics M- Monitor vital signs

| 73)

Magnesium Sulfate overdose.

"Help our babies" | **Magnesium Sulfate overdose**

This is the drug of choice for Pregnancy induced Hypertension (PIH). It is important to know the side effects of magnesium toxicity:

H - Hyporeflexia (decrease in deep tendon reflexes)

O - Oliguria (Urine output less than 30cc/hr)

B - Bradypnea (Respirations less than 12/min)

Help Our Babies (HOB) to remember the side effects of magnesium toxicity.

In essence, the magnesium sulfate is "Helping Our Babies" |
| 74)

Difference in OD, OS, and OU.

"Think S/D" | **Abbreviations used for eye drops**

Think of S/D (like Systolic/Diastolic) Hence, S is on the left and D is on the right: OD for right and OS for left.

OD is for right eye

OS is for left eye

OU is both eyes |

75) Subjective and Objective data: "*Subject is something you talk about*"	**Differences in Subjective and Objective** To remember the difference in Subjective and Objective data: Think of Subjective as a subject that you are talking about. The patient talks about a subject. Therefore, subjective data can be: complaints of pain, or a headache, or anything a patient "talks about". Objective data is something you can see: blood, results of labs, edema.

76) Signs and symptoms of IDA: "TRICEPS"	**Signs and symptoms of iron deficiency anemia** To remember the s/s of Iron deficiency anemia (IDA), use this phrase: "You may need iron for strong biceps, but, use the acronym TRICEPS." T- Tinnitus R- Red blood cell distributions width elevated (RDW elevated) I- Iron level low C- Cheilosis (lesions at corners of mouth) E- Easily fatigued P- Pallor S- Spoon-shaped finger nails
77) Causes of Aplastic anemia "CHID"	**Causes of Aplastic anemia** C- Chemical toxins H- Hepatitis I- Idiopathic causes D- Drugs: antibiotics, antiepileptic, antidiabetic.

78) Signs and symptoms of Aplastic anemia: "BLADE"	**Signs and symptoms of Aplastic anemia.** To remember the signs and symptoms of aplastic anemia use this acronym: BLADE B- Bleeding L- Low hemoglobin A- Anemia D- Dyspnea E- Ecchymoses
79) Treatment of Aplastic anemia: "PREAMP"	**Treatment of Aplastic anemia** P- Protective precautions R- Recombinant human granulocyte-macrophage colony stimulating factor (GMCSF) E- Early bone marrow transplantation A- Antibiotics/ Analgesics M- Monitor Vital signs/ and I/O P- Platelets

80) Coumadin and Heparin Antidotes: "*Think HP and CK*"	**Antidotes for Coumadin and Heparin** Think of HP (as in Hewlett-Packard) and CK (as in Calvin-Klein): *HP* -for Heparin the antidote is Protamine Sulfate *CK* -for Coumadin's antidote is Vitamin K

81)

Clinical manifestations of CVA:

"SPLASH"

Clinical manifestations of a cardiovascular accident (CVA)

To remember the clinical manifestations of a CVA use this acronym: SPLASH

S- Syncope

P- Paresthesia

L- Level of consciousness changes

A- Aphasia

S- Seizures

H- Headaches

82) Patient teaching for patients with hiatal hernia: "ACCUSE"	**Patient teaching for patients with hiatal hernia** To remember patient teaching goals for those with a hiatal hernia use this phrase: "Patients don't need an excuse when you use the acronym ACCUSE." A- Appointments: keep follow-up appointments C- Coughing should be avoided C- Constrictive clothing should be avoided U- Upright for 2 hours after eating S- Stop drinking carbonated beverages E- Eat small frequent meals

83)

Clinical manifestations of Pneumothorax :

"BAD PAST"

Clinical manifestations of Pneumothorax

To remember the signs and symptoms of Pneumothorax use this phrase:

" With pneumothorax you want the patients breathing to last; you don't want them to have a BAD PAST."

B- Breath sounds absent or diminished unilaterally

A- Anxiety

D- Dyspnea

P- Pallor

A- Atmospheric pressure in the pleural space

S- Subcutaneous emphysema

T- Tachycardia / and Tachypnea

84) Treatment of Pneumothorax: "TOPIC"	**Treatment of Pneumothorax** To remember the treatment for Pneumothorax us this phrase: "A pinprick will not cause a Pneumothorax; but, to remember how to treat it use the word TOPIC." T- Thoracentesis O- Oxygen therapy P- Position in high-fowler's I- Incentive spirometer C- Chest tube
85) Types of Pulmonary Embolism: "FAT"	**Types of Pulmonary Embolism** To remember the different types of pulmonary embolism use this acronym: FAT F- Fat A- Air T- Thrombus

86) Clinical manifestations of Pulmonary Embolism: "CHAT DATE"	**Clinical manifestations of Pulmonary Embolism** To remember the signs and symptoms of pulmonary embolism use this phrase: "CHAT with a DATE." C- Cough H- Hemoptysis A- Anxiety T- Tachypnea D- Dyspnea A- Arrhythmias T- Tachycardia E- Elevated Temperature
87) Medical treatment for Pulmonary Embolism: "FILMCLIP"	**Medical treatment for Pulmonary Embolism** To remember the medical treatment for pulmonary embolism use this phrase: "Treatment of pulmonary embolism doesn't have to be a hardship when you think of the word FILMCLIP."

F- Fibrinolytics: (urokinase, streptokinase)

I- IV therapy

L- Lab tests: (PT, PTT, ABG's)

M- Monitor I/O, VS, CVP

C- Coumadin

L- Lasix

I- Incentive spirometer

P- Position in High-fowlers

88)

Clinical manifestations of Cushing's syndrome:

"WASHRAG"

Clinical manifestations of Cushing's syndrome (hypercortisolism)

To remember the signs and symptoms of Cushing's syndrome use this phrase: "Just because Cushing's syndrome patients retain water is no need to nag; just remember the term WASHRAG."

W- Weight gain

A- Amenorrhea

S- Skin that's fragile

H - Hypertension

R- Retention of water; i.e., moon face.

A- Acne

G- Gynecomastia

89) Treatment for Cushing's syndrome: "HELP"	**Treatment for Cushing's syndrome** To remember the treatment for Cushing's syndrome use this acronym: HELP H- High potassium and high protein diet. E- Edecrin (ethacrynic acid) L- Lasix (furosemide) P- Potassium supplements
90) Hypocalcemia "3 C's"	**Hypocalcemia** Normal serum calcium: 8.5-10.5 mEq/L Think of 3 C's when assessing for hypocalcemia: C- Chvostek's sign - the patient will have facial spasms when tapping face anterior to ear. C- Cramps possible in legs, hands, and feet. C- Circumoral paraesthesia.

Topic	Tip
91) Medication for Glaucoma: "Use the car in pilocarpine to think of a car going through a tunnel"	**Medication for Glaucoma** Pilocarpine Hydrochloride is used to treat glaucoma. To remember this, use this phrase: Think of a *car going through a tunnel*; the word car is in Pilocarpine and it is used to treat the tunnel vision of Glaucoma. The slow loss of peripheral vision "tunnel vision" is caused by chronic Glaucoma and treated by Pilocarpine.
92) Difference in pronation and suppination: "Suppination- Like holding soup"	**Difference in pronation and suppination** Think of holding a bowl of *soup* when you think about *supination*. Supination is when the hand is facing up. Pronation is when the hand is facing down. The opposite of supination.

93)

Flexion and
extension:

"Flexion as in
flexing your
muscles."

**Difference in Flexion and
extension**

Flexion is when you bend a limb at
the joint; *think of flexion as "flexing
muscles"*. When you get this mental
picture in your mind, you will
remember what flexion is.

Extension is when you straighten a
limb.

94)

Abduction and
adduction:

"When
someone is
abducted,
they are taken
away"

**Difference in Abduction and
adduction**

Abduction is moving a limb away
from the midline of the body; *think
of "ab" as taking away*, like an
abduction of a person.

Adduction is moving a limb toward
the midline of the body; *think of
"Add" as adding to something*.

95)

Antidiabetics:

"DOG"

**Antidiabetics: meds used for type
2 Diabetes**

To remember oral hypoglycemic
meds used to treat diabetes Type 2
use this phrase:

"To control type 2 diabetes you
won't be in the fog when you think of
the word DOG"

	D- Diabinese (chlorpropamide) O- Orinase (glipizied) G- Glucagon (glucagen)
96) Clinical manifestations of metabolic acidosis: "CHIN"	**Clinical manifestations of metabolic acidosis** Metabolic acidosis is an acid-base imbalance resulting from excessive retention of acid or excessive excretion of HC03 To remember the signs and symptoms of metabolic acidosis use this phrase: "In metabolic acidosis the patient may have cool and clammy skin; but, to remember the signs and symptoms use the acronym CHIN." C- Cold and clammy skin / Confusion H- Headache I- Increased respiratory rate and depth N- Nausea and vomiting

97) Clinical manifestations of metabolic alkalosis: "FACT"	**Clinical manifestations of metabolic alkalosis** Metabolic alkalosis is an acid-base imbalance characterized by excessive loss of acid or excessive gain HCO3 To remember the signs and symptoms of metabolic alkalosis use this phrase: "In metabolic alkalosis the patients' fingers and toes may be intact, but remember the word FACT." F- Fingers and toes have tingling sensation A- Apnea possible; shallow respirations are more common. C- Confusion T- Tetany

98) Clinical manifestations of respiratory acidosis: "FIB"	**Clinical manifestations of respiratory acidosis** To remember the signs and symptoms of respiratory acidosis use this acronym: FIB. F- Feeling of fullness in head I- Increased pulse, and respiratory rate B- Blood pressure increased
99) Clinical manifestations of respiratory alkalosis: "PICT"	**Clinical manifestations of respiratory alkalosis** To remember the signs and symptoms of respiratory alkalosis use this phrase: "You don't have to predict convulsions; you just need to think of the word PICT. P- Positive Chvostek sign I- Inability to concentrate C-Convulsions T- Twitching of muscles

100) Procardia	**Procardia** Procardia is used for hypertension and chronic angina. One way to remember this drug is to break it into syllables: pro "meaning for" and cardia "meaning heart". Hence, procardia means "for heart".
101) Fat-Soluble Vitamins: "DEKA"	**Fat-Soluble Vitamins** Too much of fat-soluble vitamins can be toxic. To remember the fat soluable vitamins think of the prefix DEKA. It is a prefix used in the metric system. D- D Vitamin E- E Vitamin K- K Vitamin A- A Vitamin These are the fat soluble vitamins. Just remember that too much DEKA is bad for you : too much of fat-soluble vitamins is toxic.

www.ingramcontent.com/pod-product-compliance
Lightning Source LLC
Chambersburg PA
CBHW051213170526
45166CB00005B/1869